Test-Tube Conception

Test-Tube Conception

Professor Carl Wood
C.B.E., M.B.B.S., F.R.C.S., F.R.C.O.G., F.R.A.C.O.G.

Ann Westmore

A SPECTRUM BOOK

Prentice-Hall, Inc.,
Englewood Cliffs, New Jersey 07632

Library of Congress Cataloging in Publication Data

Wood, Carl.
   Test-tube conception.

   "A Spectrum Book."
   Includes index.
   1. Fertilization in vitro, Human.   I. Westmore, Ann.
II. Title.
RG135.W66   1984   618.1'78059   83-24425
ISBN 0-13-911941-8
ISBN 0-13-911909-4 (pbk.)

10 9 8 7 6 5 4 3 2 1

ISBN 0-13-911941-8

ISBN 0-13-911909-4 {PBK.}

Editorial/production supervision
and book design by Eric Newman
Cover design by Hal Siegel
Manufacturing buyer: Doreen Cavallo

Prentice-Hall International, Inc., *London*
Prentice-Hall of Australia Pty. Limited, *Sydney*
Prentice-Hall Canada Inc., *Toronto*
Prentice-Hall of India Private Limited, *New Delhi*
Prentice-Hall of Japan, Inc., *Tokyo*
Prentice-Hall of Southeast Asia Pte. Ltd., *Singapore*
Whitehall Books Limited, *Wellington, New Zealand*
Editora Prentice-Hall do Brasil Ltda., *Rio de Janeiro*

When she said I was pregnant I thought of all those wonderful things to say—thank you, you have done a wonderful job—and I just burst into tears and cried for a solid five minutes, I think, and she kept saying, "Are you all right? Are you all right?" and I just cried and cried and I think I could not believe it could ever happen to me.

Excerpt from test-tube-baby documentary film
Tomorrow's Child, Nomad Films

Contents

Acknowledgments

I wish to acknowledge the help of all those contributing to the development and success of the technique, some of whom are mentioned in Chapter 3; the dedicated scientists, technicians, and medical, nursing, and administrative staff who have enabled the procedure to be carried out; Monash and Melbourne Universities, the Queen Victoria Medical Centre, the Royal Women's Hospital, St. Andrew's Hospital, and Epworth Medical Centre, which supported the program during the difficult stage of development; research workers in the Howard Florey and Prince Henry's Hospital Research Institutes; and the Ford Foundation and the National Health and Medical Research Council of Australia for financial support.

I also wish to thank my wife, Judy, and my family, who have been understanding and patient during my involvement in the work, and my good friend Margot Corbett for her generous support.

CARL WOOD

Teams involved in the test-tube-baby programs do not make life; they assist in creation by using God's materials—the sperm cells of the husband, the egg of the wife, and the brains and skills of scientists, doctors, and many others.

Professor Carl Wood
and Ann Westmore

Introduction

The search for a cause and a successful treatment of infertility can be one of the most baffling and frustrating experiences of a lifetime. It is a search of vital importance to an estimated 10 to 15 percent of couples who are involuntarily childless. Various treatments for infertility have been devised and practiced this century. Some have been modestly successful, others counterproductive.

In recent years, many couples with infertility problems have had new hope following the development of what has become known as "the test-tube-baby procedure." In essence, this involves the exposure of the human egg to sperm cells in the laboratory (*in vitro* fertilization: IVF) and the transfer of the resulting embryo to the mother's uterus (embryo transfer: ET).

The test-tube-baby procedure is not a panacea. It does not cure infertility, but to a significant proportion of couples with infertility problems it offers the possibility of bypassing a barrier to conception.

After three treatment attempts, at least four out of ten couples who join the program can expect to achieve a pregnancy.

Couples who join an IVF program may suffer feelings of sadness, helplessness, anger, and frustration, but above all a devastating sense of emptiness.

At first glance, infertility (a defect) plus the test-tube-baby procedure (a treatment) may result in a child. Such oversimplification may light a flame of hope but ignores so much that lies between—all the time and effort involved in the procedure, the stress, pain, skill, and determination.

Some of those who have been through a treatment attempt liken it to a particularly difficult obstacle race, the difference being that if one falls in an obstacle race it is possible to get up and continue,

1

sometimes even to win. In the obstacle race of an IVF attempt, any fall at any time signifies the failure of that attempt. It is only natural that couples become upset—even angry—if something goes wrong.

There are many steps, and many opportunities for human error, in the complicated test-tube-baby procedure, and team members are not infallible. If couples feel that they, after having cooperated in every possible way, have been let down by the team, their disappointment and frustration may be acute.

The IVF method of conception is obviously much more complex than the natural system. And it is difficult to predict which couples will be able to meet the demands and uncertainties involved.

Because mutual support, understanding, and the ability to cope are important elements in the partnership of couples contemplating the procedure, and because communities considering its use may be the focus of intense discussion of the moral, legal, and financial aspects, a realistic understanding of IVF and ET is most important. This book was written in an attempt to increase that understanding.

The effort that IVF couples—and indirectly, communities—put into the attempts to achieve pregnancy is very significant. The test-tube-baby procedure is sometimes said to be "inhuman" because it is scientific and differs markedly from the orthodox method of conception, but the extra effort required of couples who take part in IVF programs adds a new dimension of human endeavor to the achievement of a pregnancy that compensates for the unconventional and scientific aspect. In terms of the equation of humanity and inhumanity, surely this deep and sustained application of human effort more than compensates for the unconventional and scientific aspects of the program.

A further aspect of the test-tube-baby procedure requires careful consideration. Clearly the IVF procedure is now a practical method of treating certain types of infertility. Its development, however, has far greater implications. Until recently, medicine was restricted to preventing and treating disease. It is now possible to assist in the creation of human beings. This has social and ethical consequences that are discussed in this book.

In the final analysis, the children whom the test-tube-baby procedure will help make possible—some of whom may one day read this book—will know that they were much loved and much wanted before they came into existence.

1

How Does Pregnancy Occur?

Pregnancy follows the union of an egg and a sperm cell, usually brought together by means of coitus, the act of sexual intercourse. This is the simple explanation of a very complex achievement that may be influenced and affected by any one or more of a range of psychological, social, and physical factors.

People want to have children for a variety of reasons. Some may wish to re-create themselves, others to experience the pleasure of creating a new being or of watching a child grow and develop.

Couples seeking admission to the IVF program often say that they want children for companionship, or even to play with. Others state that they wish to have children to love. Occasionally some even appear to want a child that they can dominate or direct and have already planned its life before it is born. For some men and women, pregnancy and child rearing are regarded as innate; they come with marriage and a home. Others see children as a stabilizing influence on a relationship or a means of expanding their horizons.

Undoubtedly some couples are influenced by peer-group pressures; it is a common expectation to marry and have children. Less often, a couple may want children to take over the family business, property, or inheritance.

Some parents with one child feel that they ought to have another. This is based on the popular view that the single child is spoiled or in some way deprived. Recent studies show differences between single children and children from larger families, but they do not confirm that the differences are necessarily deleterious. The single child is often more mature, outgoing, and at ease with adults, but he or she need not be a "loner." The need for playmates can be met by encouraging friendships with other youngsters.

3

Many couples in the Western world now have only two children, whereas at the beginning of the century the average number of children in countries such as Australia was five. This rapid reduction in family size stems from a variety of social and economic factors, including changing expectations such as better education for each child, the likelihood that women will have other roles besides child bearing, and increased wealth. The availability of a wide range of birth-control methods has helped transform these expectations into reality.

Family size is influenced increasingly by factors beyond the home, such as social and economic pressures. In a number of countries, in an effort to overcome chronic shortages of food and shelter, small families are actively encouraged and having a large number of children may be considered irresponsible.

Religious influences, although their impact is not always clear-cut, may also play a part in planning a family. The average family size of Roman Catholics in most Western nations is still larger than that of non-Catholics.

Conflicting views about reproduction are evident within, for example, the Christian religion. In this regard it is interesting to compare the overt anti-sexual attitudes of St. Paul (who thought it better to remain chaste) and St. Augustine (who renounced sexuality) with the pro-natal views of latter-day theologians and the high value they place on monogamy and the family unit.

Unfortunately, this ambivalence has never been resolved satisfactorily, and many couples are unable to embrace sexuality in the same positive manner that they regard the rearing of children.

Although it is well recognized that many factors influence couples to have one or several children, it is worth considering why an increasing number of people are choosing to have no children.

Social and psychological factors may operate to deter couples from becoming parents. Some decide not to have children because of foreseeable restrictions on career and leisure activities. Others may feel that getting to know and enjoy each other fully precludes spending two decades or more rearing children. The cost of feeding, clothing, and educating children is substantial and may present great difficulties for some couples, particularly in an era of high unemployment.

People may have ideological reasons for not rearing a family; some feel that the world's population is excessive already, and that world resources are stretched to the limit. Voluntary sterilization may therefore seem an attractive, and possibly responsible, proposition.

Fear and anxiety about pregnancy and childrearing may also be influential in restricting the family size. Will my child be normal?

Can I cope with pregnancy and birth? Will my body change and become less attractive? How will the pregnancy affect my marriage and sex life? Have I the ability to become a satisfactory parent?

These are questions that most would-be parents consider. And those couples already having difficulty in coping with everyday life may have reasons for anxiety about whether they can handle the additional emotional and physical demands of pregnancy, birth, and child rearing.

Many of the fears and anxieties concerning pregnancy and birth can be overcome by information and counseling, and it is increasingly a matter of personal choice and serious consideration as to whether there should be children and, if so, when.

Careful assessment of the kaleidoscope of motivational factors is important, for it brings to the surface expectations about what children can and cannot bring to a relationship.

Infertility may provide time for coming to grips with whether, and why, children are seen as desirable.

Physical factors are usually a couple's first consideration once partners have decided to have a family.

For couples wanting a child, the hope is dashed—at least temporarily—when menstruation or blood loss occurs in the menstrual cycle. The immediate reaction of the woman, and sometimes her partner also, may be one of depression, anger, frustration, and certainly disappointment.

The inability to conceive provokes many questions. Is our timing right? Are we having sex too often or too infrequently? Would it be better in another position? Is he holding back so that I won't get pregnant? Does she really have her heart in it—is she really trying?

It is not uncommon for one partner to become dissatisfied with the other, projecting his or her disappointment.

Clearly, couples need to know what is and what is not important, so that there can be a more factual approach to attempting conception without disruption of relationships.

In this connection it is useful for couples to be aware that they can time intercourse to increase the chances of a pregnancy's occurring. The key to maximizing the likelihood of pregnancy is to aim to have intercourse during those days when the woman is fertile. These are the days around the time when an egg is released from the ovary (ovulation). The body gives various signals of this event. In many women, the mucus seen at the vaginal opening is slippery and wet and resembles the white of an egg; body temperature also rises around the time of ovulation (see Chapter 5 for a guide to measuring daily temperature).

Some couples seek counseling for infertility. Closer questioning often reveals that one of the partners is sabotaging the effort to become pregnant.

The male partner may do this by exhausting himself with his work or leisure activities, always being incapable of having intercourse at the fertile time of the menstrual cycle. Or the female may complain of tiredness, headache, or difficulty in defining the fertile part of the cycle. Excuses used in avoiding intercourse may not become apparent until a detailed account of the sexual history is taken. In this situation, subconscious factors may help to explain why the partner involved does not want a pregnancy.

Sexual union is instinctual in all species and is influenced by hormonal and emotional factors. It is not the purpose of this book to explore the whole area of human sexuality; but anxiety concerning sexuality, derived either from childhood or early adult experiences, is the most usual factor responsible for sexual impairment.

Physical causes of sexual dysfunction, which are discussed in more detail in Chapter 2, can be diagnosed by medical assessment, and treatment is available for many types of disorder. However, this often requires time and patience, both on the part of the couple and their counselor.

Normally, when a woman is sexually aroused, a number of well-documented changes occur that help to make intercourse pleasurable and effective and that tend to favor conception.

For example, sexual excitement increases secretion through the lining cells of the vagina, which facilitates movement of the penis. Some of the discomfort occurring during intercourse is related to un-readiness of the female to accept the penis, so loving preparation for intercourse is very important. Coincident with increased secretion, the vagina alters in shape so that the penis is more readily accepted without discomfort; while the upper part of the vagina enlarges, the lower part constricts, the vagina becoming pear-shaped.

Accompanying the changing shape of the vagina and the increased secretion, the uterus moves upward out of the pelvis, and, in doing so, the ovaries are supported away from the moving penis, which otherwise might cause pain during intercourse.

The semen (the male ejaculate containing sperm cells) comes to lie in a pool close to the cervix (the neck of the uterus) so that the sperm cells have ready access to the uterus and Fallopian tubes (see Figure 1).

For the male to contribute satisfactorily to conception, three

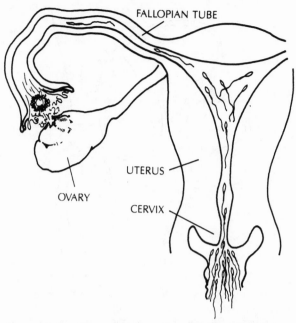

FALLOPIAN TUBE

UTERUS

OVARY

CERVIX

Figure 1. Ovulation: the egg, surrounded by smaller, sticky cells, passes from a follicle in the ovary to the Fallopian tube. Sperm move through the vagina and the uterus to meet the egg in the tube.

major factors are required: adequate production of semen, the ability to erect the penis, and a satisfactory ejaculation.

The sperm cells are manufactured in two testicles (the testes) as a result of hormones' (chemical messenger substances) passing to them from the brain via the bloodstream (see Figure 2).

For conception to occur, the semen must be of a satisfactory quality. Information about the most favorable characteristics of semen required for conception is still incomplete, and sometimes pregnancy occurs when the male partner is thought to be infertile. On the other hand, men who appear to be highly fertile may never become fathers.

The two most important qualities of the semen that are known to be related to male fertility potential are the number of sperm cells that the semen contains and the activity of the sperm cells.

Sperm counts of more than 20 million per milliliter and normal motility (that is, 50 to 70 percent of the sperm cells are active when examined under the microscope) are considered satisfactory.

Less commonly, other qualities of the semen may affect fertility or indicate reduced fertility. For example, the total volume of the

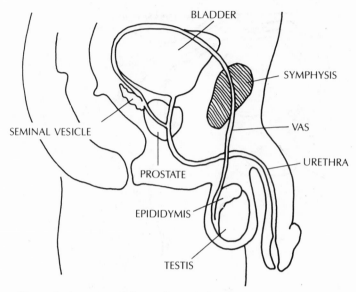

Figure 2. Anatomy of the male genital organs: sperm are produced in the testes and pass along the vas and urethra to the end of the penis. Extra fluid and chemicals may be added to the semen by the epididymis, seminal vesicles, and prostate.

ejaculate may be substantially below normal, a large proportion of the sperm cells may have an abnormal appearance when examined under the microscope, or the semen may be infected or may lack certain chemical substances.

The average ejaculate contains between 20 million and 300 million sperm cells. The reason for such a large number is in part related to the relatively long and hazardous journey to be completed before a sperm cell can gain access to the egg. In fact, only about 100 sperm cells ever reach even the vicinity of the egg, and by virtue of the journey they must make, probably only the fittest travel the length of a Fallopian tube.

The large number of sperm cells in the average ejaculate is, in some ways, a fail-safe measure for continuation of the human species. Should some environmental factor reduce sperm counts, there would still be a sufficient abundance to sustain male fertility, except in men with borderline counts.

Erection of the penis depends on emotional arousal and a system of messages sent from the brain to the penis whereby blood is trapped within it, ensuring its hardness. This allows the introduction of the penis into the vagina. Some men have no difficulty obtaining an erection but, on attempting to introduce the penis into the vagina, the erection disappears. This may be caused by anxiety concerning intercourse itself—thus impeding the passage of messages from the brain to the penis. Skilled counseling and behavioral treatment may prove helpful.

During ejaculation, sperm cells are propelled into the vagina, accompanied by a feeling of excitement and release. Some men who have an erect penis cannot ejaculate into the vagina, while in others incomplete ejaculation may occur. When these problems are caused by emotional factors they can usually be overcome by counseling. An alternative is for the semen to be placed in the partner's vagina after masturbation.

Physical disorders may also prevent effective ejaculation, and treatment may help if the condition is reversible.

The journey of the sperm cells through the female genital tract is dependent partly on the activity of the sperm cells themselves, and partly on female factors. The sperm cells swim by mean of a tail, and their activity viewed under the microscope is similar to that of a tadpole.

Movement of the sperm cells is affected by the thickness or viscosity of the fluid in the female genital tract, the muscular activity of the walls of the uterus and Fallopian tubes, and the current in the tubes created by fine hairlike structures called *cilia*, which beat rapidly in one direction or the other.

Undoubtedly, the activity of the sperm cells aids their passage, but it is unclear how important the female factors mentioned above are in enhancing or inhibiting the migration of the sperm cells through the Fallopian tubes.

In order for fertilization to occur, a ripe egg (also called the *ovum*) must pass from the ovary into a Fallopian tube (Figure 1).

Approximately once each month, a small crop of eggs develops in the ovary within tiny cysts of fluid called *follicles*. From this crop of eggs, one is selected to be the ripe follicle of the month. When fully mature, the egg is surrounded by a gel-like coat and a layer of cells that assists in its development; and this whole mass is contained within a follicle about two centimeters in diameter.

The ripening of the egg and of the cells surrounding it is stimulated by hormones produced within the ovary. The most important hormone involved in egg ripening is Estrogen. The manufacture of Estrogen in the ovary is under the control of another hormone—Follicle Stimulating Hormone—manufactured within the pituitary gland, a small structure at the base of the brain.

The ovary and the pituitary gland work together, sending hormones back and forth in order to coordinate the ripening of the follicle and egg.

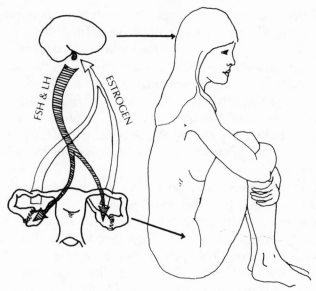

Figure 3. Ovulation and menstruation depend upon chemical messengers (LH and FSH) sent from the brain to stimulate production of hormones (Estrogen and Progesterone) in the ovary. Ovarian hormones affect egg ripening, ovulation, and menstruation.

By measuring the hormones produced by the pituitary gland and the ovary, scientists have been able to study the sequence of egg ripening in some detail.

The hormones that stimulate egg development and release are called *pituitary gonadotropins*. There are two of these—Follicle Stimulating Hormone (FSH), which, as the name suggests, spurs development of a follicle and the egg within, and Luteinizing Hormone (LH), which completes the final development of the egg and triggers its release once it is ripe (the process of ovulation).

The LH level in the bloodstream increases rapidly about one day before ovulation, and this chemical message determines the time at which the egg will leave the follicle and pass into the Fallopian tube.

The exact mechanism whereby the egg leaves the follicle within the ovary is uncertain, but both physical and chemical factors are known to be involved. The pressure in the follicle increases so that the small cyst bursts and the egg gently floats from it. Before this happens, chemical changes weaken the wall of the follicle, thus making eruption of the small balloon easier.

When the egg leaves the ovary, it is surrounded by a mass of cells that are held together by a sticky material. The sticky nature of this material helps the egg to adhere to the fimbriae (the fringe-like processes at the end of the Fallopian tube that slide over the ovary). In this way the egg passes into the tube, instead of being lost within the abdomen.

When the egg passes into the tube, it does not take an active role in its own transport. Rather, it relies on the activity of the fine cilia that line the tube, and on the muscular contractions of the tube, for its propulsion. If the ripe egg meets sperm cells in the tube, fertilization may occur. The precise length of time that the egg can remain healthy in the tube awaiting the sperm cells is uncertain, but it is probably at least twelve to twenty-four hours.

Before a sperm cell can pass into the egg, it has to penetrate the outer coat of the egg. This is achieved by dissolving the outer coat material by means of chemical reactions involving substances from the sperm cell and the Fallopian tube. The substances contributed by the sperm cell to this process are made available during "capacitation"— a change, involving the shedding of part of the sperm cell head, that occurs as the sperm cell passes through the genital tract. The penetration of the sperm cell into the egg is also aided by its own physical activity.

As soon as one sperm cell has penetrated the outer coat, chemicals released from the interior of the egg pass to the coat, where they help create a chemical barrier to the entry of further sperm cells.

If more than one sperm cell enters the egg, fertilization and subsequent embryo development may fail or be abnormal.

Once a sperm cell has penetrated the egg—which may take only one to two hours in the laboratory—the process of fertilization is under way. Genetic material from the sperm cell and the egg is rearranged, and within about twelve to eighteen hours male and female genetic material is apparent under the microscope as clumps within the fertilized egg. The fertilized egg is now called a *one-cell embryo*.

Following this, a series of simple divisions start: into two cells, then four, then eight, and so on. Each early cell division takes about twelve hours.

A two-cell embryo has formed by approximately twenty-four hours, a four-cell embryo by about thirty-six hours, a sixteen-cell embryo by about three days. Fertilization and development of the embryo occur in the Fallopian tube, and by the time the embryo has developed to about the eight- to sixteen-cell stage, it has reached the uterus.

It is another three days before the embryo embeds in the nutritive lining of the uterus, which is known as the *endometrium*. During this three-day wait in the uterus, the embryo undergoes further growth, and fluid appears within it. At this stage, it is referred to as a *blastocyst*,

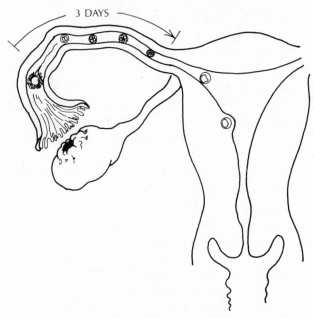

Figure 4. Egg is fertilized by sperm in segment of tube closest to the ovary. Fertilized egg develops to an eight- to sixteen-cell embryo over three days as it passes down the tube to the uterus. The embryo spends two to three days in the uterus, where it divides further into many more cells before embedding in the wall of the uterus.

and it contains three basic structures: a thin layer of cells around the outside that will subsequently form the placenta and the membrane surrounding the baby; an inner mass of cells that is destined to form the organs of the baby; and, in between, fluid that will cushion the fetus and act as a chemical store during its development.

The implantation of the blastocyst in the endometrium is not clearly understood. Evidence suggests that the process may involve some form of chemical and physical interaction between the blastocyst and the endometrium, the endometrium being dissolved and also engulfing the blastocyst.

The life of the early embryo and fetus is sustained by the continued activity of the follicle in the ovary from which the egg has come. In particular, this follicle (now called the *corpus luteum*) produces Pro- gesterone, which helps prepare the nutritive endometrium.

2

Questions About Infertility

Couples and others interested in the procedure often have many questions about infertility. The questions most often asked are dealt with in this chapter.

What is infertility? —

Infertility refers to an inability to conceive, but the term has some elasticity, as a couple may appear to be infertile for a year or more and then conceive.

Subfertility is the term sometimes used to described a reduced state of fertility. In such cases some factor or factors, such as a low sperm count or the blockage of a Fallopian tube, reduce the chance of conception's occurring.

Sterility means that one can never conceive unless some form of medical intervention occurs.

How is infertility defined?

If couples are unable to conceive after one year of regular sexual intercourse, a doctor may diagnose a state of infertility. The reason for choosing one year is that 85 to 90 percent of couples become pregnant within this time, many after four to five months of regular intercourse.

This medical definition of infertility may sometimes be unsatisfactory. A person may already be aware of factors—such as previous surgery, prior pregnancy, or a previous infection in the pelvis—that have reduced his or her fertility, and these factors should be taken into account when determining whether examination and investigation of infertility are warranted.

An estimated 10 to 15 percent of couples in many western countries are infertile or subfertile.

Is there any evidence that infertility is becoming more prevalent?

Yes, there is evidence that this is so.

In some studies, average sperm counts in males appear to have declined in the past two decades, and the increased number of patients attending infertility clinics may be another indication of a growing problem.

A number of factors, some of which are discussed in the following section, may have contributed to an increased incidence of infertility.

The use of the intrauterine device (IUD) has resulted occasionally in infection of and irreversible damage to the Fallopian tubes. The use of the Pill (in place of the condom, which acts as a barrier to the sexually transmitted organisms that may cause infertility) and increased sexual permissiveness may have resulted in an increased risk of venereal disease—an important cause of infertility. Fortunately, this effect has been ameliorated to some extent by improved treatment of venereal diseases with antibiotics.

The greater availability of abortion—both legal and illegal—may have resulted in a greater incidence of infertility either because of infection of the Fallopian tubes or because of damage to the cervix resulting in an inability to maintain the pregnancy.

The trend to postpone the first pregnancy may contribute to the occurrence of infertility, for while delaying the starting of a family, a woman has the usual risk of developing pelvic infection or endometriosis, a condition in which the endometrium grows in areas of the pelvis other than the uterus.

Other factors that may be contributing to an *apparent* increase in infertility are:

- the rapid expansion of the treatment of infertility as a specialist branch of medicine has increased awareness that expert help and improved treatments are available;
- the greater need to overcome problems of infertility (because of the declining number of babies available for adoption) may have encouraged

14

couples to come forward; and a general acceptance of more open discussion about pregnancy and infertility problems has reduced embarrassment about seeking medical advice and assistance: even twenty or thirty years ago, many couples were reluctant to discuss apparent infertility, as most aspects of reproduction were not matters of polite—or even intimate—conversation.

Why treat infertility?

It is sometimes argued that the treatment of infertility is unimportant because there are too many children in the world already.

This may be true in a global sense, and the resolution of problems of overpopulation, malnutrition, and conservation of world resources is very important.

However, it ignores the extreme anguish and distress of couples who cannot have children. Even in overpopulated societies, the inability to conceive often causes great concern.

The World Health Organization has stated that every couple has the right to establish a family and has backed this view with support for research into the causes and treatment of infertility.

The resolution of infertility problems has many important implications. To begin with, it may contribute to the improved emotional health of many couples. The losses arising from infertility are often invisible to others but enormously real and distressing to those who are affected. It is not unusual for people with an infertility problem to feel that they have lost the chance to experience conception, pregnancy, and birth; the opportunity to give the gift of a grandchild to their own parents; the potential for a shared part in the creation of an individual. They may cry often, feel numb, sad, anxious, restless, angry, resentful; retrace past events again and again as they mourn the loss of the family they may have planned or dreamed about.

Another reason for treating infertility is in the interests of a particular nation. For example, where government policies rely on population growth and where 10 to 15 percent of the population is infertile, it would seem compatible with the national interest to treat infertility. Government policies, for example, are often based on a predicted population increase. Obviously, in countries where policies rely on a stabilizing of population numbers, the reverse may be true.

One argument put forward by those opposed to treating infertility is that infertile couples are "less fit" than the general population. Therefore—the argument goes—it would be best if they did not reproduce and perpetuate problems of infertility.

15

This argument raises two questions. First, are infertile couples any less fit emotionally, intellectually, or even physically than the rest of the population?

This is the subject of some dispute. Clearly, the infertile person has a physical disorder, but so too do people with asthma, arthritis, or diabetes, and no one suggests that such people should not attempt to have children. And certainly there is no evidence that intellectual deficiency is related to infertility. Emotional problems—if they occur at all—tend to be caused by the problem of infertility, rather than the reverse. Indeed, most doctors treating infertile couples consider that their similarities to the general population are much greater than any difference.

The second question concerns the extent to which infertility is an inherited disorder, so that by treating it, one is perpetuating problems for the next generation.

Very few known causes of infertility are of a genetic nature, and thus it would be unlikely for an infertility problem to be handed down from generation to generation. Diseased Fallopian tubes, for example, are a major cause of infertility but are certainly not inherited. Hormonal problems in men and women do not usually have a genetic basis, and many cases of sperm disorders are caused by noninheritable birth defects such as undescended testes or hormone deficiencies or by accidents. Others argue against treating infertility on the basis of cost/benefit analyses of the available treatments. Financial aspects of IVF treatment are discussed in detail in Chapters 6 and 9.

When do most couples see a doctor if they are worried about fertility?

Most couples seek advice after six to twelve months of trying unsuccessfully to conceive.

Some do not wait this long. They may have decided to start a family soon after marriage, or they may have married in their late thirties or early forties and wish to have a child as soon as possible. Other couples wait several years before seeking medical advice. Initially, such couples may have considered children unimportant and later changed their minds, or they became curious about why a pregnancy had not occurred.

Some couples see a doctor before marriage to ensure that both partners are potentially fertile. If fertility is considered to be an essential aspect of marriage, it is desirable that any problem concerning fertility be detected prior to marriage so that disappointment in this regard is known before a commitment is made.

Is there anything we can do to aid conception?

A state of good general health is thought to be important. However, since fertility rates in many specific groups of people are high despite large differences in physical and emotional health, and as conception occurs at least as frequently following rape as in the natural situation, it is difficult to argue the importance of general physical and psychological health.

Fatigue in one or both partners sometimes contributes to infertility— usually by reducing the frequency of sexual activity. Partners who are involved in careers that require considerable travel may have difficulty conceiving. And often a pregnancy does not occur until lifestyles are more settled.

Excessive weight gain or loss should be avoided if pregnancy is desired. Numerous studies have linked significant weight changes with an absence of menstrual periods, indicating that ovulation is not occurring and therefore pregnancy is impossible.

An adequate intake of trace elements and vitamins is thought to be important for fertility, on the basis of research studies on animals. Assuming a balanced diet, specific mineral deficiencies are unlikely to occur in most countries.

Smoking and drinking may alter fertility, but this is not proven. Some substances in smoke can affect the genital tract; for example, nicotine alters the activity of the uterus, and, theoretically, this could influence conception. In sensitive individuals, nicotine or any of the hundreds of other substances contained in smoke could have a specific anti-fertility effect. Certainly, smoking does hasten the advent of meno- pause, so in this sense, the number of fertile years is reduced. Like smoke constituents, alcohol has effects on the genital tract. For example, it blocks uterine activity. Excessive amounts of alcohol may also depress the nervous system and produce impotence (inability to achieve penile erection). However, some of the effects of alcohol may be favorable: it reduces anxiety about sexual performance in some people and so may make it easier for the male partner to sustain an erection.

For couples seeking assistance and in whom no other cause of infertility is found, it is probably worthwhile not to smoke or to drink alcohol for four to six months. Should a pregnancy occur, such lifestyle changes are known to be beneficial to the developing child.

Marijuana may inhibit ejaculation in the male, and heavy marijuana smokers should be aware of this.

Various types of medication may affect fertility, and it is worthwhile asking your doctor if any drugs you are taking could be harmful to fertility. In some women taking anti-depressant drugs there may be excessive production of the hormone Prolactin. This tends to suppress ovulation and stimulate milk production. However, the question of taking these drugs is not clear cut, as some people may become sexually potent as a result of resolution of anxiety and depression.

Recent publicity about jogging has suggested that women joggers may experience hormonal changes and failure to ovulate. Excessive exercise may be associated with marked weight loss resulting in suppression of ovulation. On the other hand, many people feel better and experience increased libido when they are fit. Insofar as regular exercise may produce a feeling of well-being and increased libido, it may be a self-help measure worth trying.

Can we treat ourselves for infertility?

Women can help themselves to some extent by determining whether they are ovulating. This can be checked by noting temperature each day during the menstrual cycle (see Chapter 5 for instructions) and/ or by checking the mucus changes evident at the vaginal opening.

In addition to determining whether ovulation is occuring, it is important to find out when it occurs. The chances of conception are maximized by matching the time of intercourse with the time of ovulation.

Unfortunately, neither the mucus changes nor the temperature rise is an exact indicator of the time of ovulation. The temperature rise may occur one day before or after ovulation, and similarly the occurrence of the last day of lubricative, stretchy "fertile-type" mucus only approximates ovulation.

For this reason couples who have regular intercourse during the most fertile week of the cycle are as likely to achieve a pregnancy as they would be if they tried to time intercourse to coincide precisely with the mucus and temperature markers of ovulation. This approach of regular intercourse during the fertile week suits many couples, as they do not need to measure temperature each day, nor do they feel quite as compelled to have intercourse on a particular day.

In general, sexual behavior is an important factor in determining the likelihood of conception: couples who have intercourse four times a week conceive in about one-third the time of those having intercourse once a week.

Couples who have infrequent intercourse or who are producing the fertile-type mucus only rarely may prefer the approach of charting mucus and/or temperature changes.

If I am ovulating and am having intercourse during the fertile phase but am still not pregnant, what should I do?

At this stage you would be wise to seek medical assistance.

Most patients initially see their general practitioner (GP), who is likely to do several simple tests to try to determine the cause of the problem. For example, the GP often arranges for a semen analysis together with mucus and temperature checks to assess whether ovulation is occurring. It is important for men having a semen analysis to follow carefully the instructions they are given; otherwise the result can be misleading.

Some doctors also arrange for an X ray to determine whether the uterus and tubes are normal, and a curettage (endometrial biopsy) may be performed also. The latter involves microscopic examination of a scraping from the endometrium in the second half of a monthly cycle. This enables assessment of the influence of the hormone Progesterone on the endometrium. Adequate levels of Progesterone are essential both for implantation of the embryo and for the creation of an environment that encourages early development.

If the cause of infertility is not apparent, or there is a possible cause that requires further investigation, referral to a specialist is advisable. The specialist will take a history and carry out a physical examination of both partners. Then various investigations will probably be required to determine the cause or causes of infertility.

Frequently the cause is not obvious from the history and physical examination. For example, only about one in two patients with diseased Fallopian tubes has a history suggesting its presence. Thus couples nearly always have to undergo a series of tests, and generally the commonly known causes of infertility are investigated first.

What is involved in an adequate initial screening for infertility problems?

Doctors vary in the type and number of tests they use in attempts to diagnose the cause of infertility, and it is therefore reasonable to have a checklist of what would constitute a thorough investigation.

19

A reasonable workup includes three semen analyses, ovulation tests, female hormone measurements (both Progesterone and Prolactin), a post-coital test, a laparoscopy, and a curettage.

How long does it take to assess a couple's state of fertility?

The need for several semen analyses as well as other investigations of both partners means that it may take several months to pinpoint the cause of infertility. Assessment may extend beyond this if the cause of the infertility is uncommon or if no apparent cause can be found.

If couples have limited time in which to establish the cause of infertility and to start treatment, they should make their position clear to the doctor so that arrangements can be made to do several investigations simultaneously. This approach may have the disadvantage of requiring additional tests and expense, but this should be weighed against the benefits of having a diagnosis sooner than it might otherwise be achieved.

What are the major events of conception at the cellular level?

First, a mature egg must make its way from the ovary into the Fallopian tube, and during the next twelve hours or so, sperm cells must arrive after journeying from the vagina.

As soon as an egg and a sperm cell have united, the embryo so formed must travel back through the tube to the uterus, arriving when both it and the endometrium are in a suitable stage of development to allow for subsequent implantation and growth.

What are the common physical causes of infertility in men, and how are they diagnosed?

Poor sperm quality and inability to ejaculate are the most usual causes.

A number of disorders may result in poor sperm quality. Sometimes the testes or other male genital organs that contribute to the semen (the male ejaculate) are improperly formed so that mature sperm cells are not produced. In the case of a male child born with undescended testes, for example, unless the testes are relocated to the scrotum at an early age, permanent damage occurs and sperm quality is never satisfactory.

A semen analysis may show oligospermia (a decreased number of sperm cells), aspermia (the absence of sperm), or sperm with reduced motility (movement).

Sometimes the organs forming the sperm cells or the tubes necessary for delivery of the sperm to the penis are blocked. Sometimes the testes or other genital organs may be damaged because of an infection. A common example of such an infection is the virus of mumps, which may affect the testes. Men who have had mumps usually do not suffer impaired sperm production, but if swelling of the scrotum occurs at the time of mumps, then permanent damage may result. Accidents or wartime wounds may be another cause of sperm abnormalities.

Hormonal abnormalities may also cause poor sperm production. The manufacture of sperm cells is under the control of hormones, which pass from the pituitary gland at the base of the brain to the testes. Precise control of sperm production is possible because of a feedback system in which substances produced in the testes pass back through the bloodstream to the pituitary gland. If the pituitary hormones are not produced in sufficient quantities, or the testes are not responsive, then the production of mature sperm cells is adversely affected.

The presence of cancer or other growths in the testes or elsewhere is a cause of impaired sperm production. This is because the anti-cancer drugs used during treatment damage the sperm-producing cells of the testes. Therefore it is now accepted medical practice to collect and freeze some sperm cells prior to treatment with anti-cancer drugs. Then if a child is desired later, this may be achieved by artificial insemination after thawing of the husband's sperm cells.

Another type of infertility in men results from the sterilization procedure vasectomy. Although vasectomy reversal is often successful in surgical terms, the quality of sperm cells after reversal may be unsatisfactory. Because of this, men who have been sterilized should be advised that reversal may not succeed, and before they decide to have a vasectomy, serious consideration should be given to having some sperm cells frozen. About 1 percent of men who are sterilized request a reversal, usually after the death of a child or following re-marriage.

Three semen analyses are usually required to diagnose a problem of consistently poor sperm quality or quantity. This is because results of semen analyses may vary according to the particular circumstances of the sperm cell collection.

A semen analysis involves abstinence from intercourse for thirty-six to forty-eight hours, followed by masturbation into a sterile jar. The sample is analyzed for sperm number, motility (movement), morphology (appearance of the sperm cells), volume of the ejaculate, and chemical constituents. If the semen analyses indicate that sperm cells are poor in quantity or quality, further investigations are carried out to determine the cause of the problem. These investigations may involve tests, examinations, and X rays for abnormalities or blockages to the tubes of the male reproductive tract. Blood samples may be taken in order to check levels of hormones involved in sperm cell production. This may provide insights into the presence of abnormalities associated with poorly developed testes.

Sometimes the sperm-producing cells of the testes need to be examined, and for this purpose a doctor performs a "needle biopsy." This enables an assessment of the cells responsible for sperm production, and, if immature sperm cells are being produced, the biopsy specimen indicates to what stage they are maturing.

If infection of the prostate gland is suspected as a cause of poor sperm quality, this gland may be examined. To do this, the doctor massages prostatic fluid from the gland by pressing the prostate gland gently with a finger in the rectum.

Apart from the health or otherwise of the sperm cells, the ability to ejaculate is an important factor in achieving a pregnancy. This ability is difficult to assess. Any laboratory analysis of the semen requires the man to ejaculate a sample into a jar. However, the stress of masturbating in the laboratory may adversely affect the ejaculation performance. Also, intercourse occurs under a variety of conditions, and ejaculation may be less effective in association with anxiety, fatigue, marijuana, or excess alcohol.

Ineffective ejaculation is of no importance if it is an occasional occurrence, but if it occurs repeatedly it can result in infertility.

What are the most usual physical causes of infertility in women, and how are they diagnosed?

More is known about the causes of female infertility, and treatment is more often successful, than it is with males.

The most common single cause of infertility in women is disease of or damage to the Fallopian tubes, estimated to account for 25 to 35 percent of cases. Any scarring of or damage to the delicate lining of the Fallopian tubes may affect the passage of the sperm cells, egg, or embryo, making a pregnancy unlikely, if not impossible.

Tubal disease is usually caused by infection occurring after birth, abortion, appendicitis, or sexual activity. Less commonly, it can occur after menstruation or if an infection is transferred from elsewhere on the body, such as a boil on the buttocks. On rare occasions infection has resulted from waterskiing when water carrying infective bacteria has been forced from the vagina into the uterus and tubes. Infection may follow surgery, particularly when disorders such as appendicitis or peritonitis have led to infection in the pelvis.

Unfortunately, many tubal infections occur without the woman's being aware of any problem. By the time treatment for infertility is sought, permanent damage to the Fallopian tubes may have occurred. Naturally, such women are curious—and often anxious—about the cause, as they are unaware of any previous problem.

Sometimes tubal disease is suspected after a physical examination, or on the basis of the individual's history. A tubal infection treated previously may provide a clue, but frequently tubal problems are not apparent until a special test is done.

The X ray or hysterosalpingogram is one investigation that enables the doctor to assess whether the tubes are blocked or whether abnormalities of the uterine cavity exist. It provides important information in deciding whether surgery would be helpful and the type of surgery that should be performed.

It is carried out in the X-ray department, and initially the doctor uses a speculum, a special instrument designed to fit into the vagina. This enables the doctor to view the cervix and to attach a tube to it through which a dye is injected. As the dye passes through the uterus and Fallopian tubes, it provides a clear X-ray picture that the woman herself can observe if a screen is placed next to her. If the tubes are blocked the fluid will not pass into the abdomen, and this is clear from the X-ray picture. This test has the advantage of not requiring an anaesthetic, and sometimes it clears the tubes of blockages. However, it may be painful, and occasionally, during or after this X ray, an allergic response or symptoms of infection may occur. Therefore, if discomfort associated with the procedure occurs, a doctor should be consulted immediately. Patients should be aware that occasionally the hysterosalpingogram may falsely indicate tubal disease as a result of tubal spasm during the procedure. A second investigation is the laparoscopy.

This surgical procedure, enabling visual inspection of the ovaries, uterus, tubes, and neighboring organs, including the outside of the bowel and bladder, can help in the diagnosis of fibroids, adhesions, endometriosis (all of which are described later in this chapter), and tubal disease.

The procedure is carried out most often under a general anaesthetic and involves two small incisions, one through the navel (umbilicus), through which is passed a combination eyepiece and light that allows the surgeon to see inside the abdomen, and the second along the hairline at the base of the abdomen through which a forceps is inserted that is used to move the uterus, tubes, or ovaries into view.

While the tubes are in view, another doctor passes a dye through the cervix into the uterus and tubes, and it is possible for the surgeon to watch the dye flow through the tubes into the abdomen. The surgeon can see precisely where blockages occur and can also get some idea of the general health of the tubes.

Laparoscopy is more reliable than the hysterosalpingogram, but it has the disadvantage of usually requiring a general anaesthetic, which may entail a slight risk. This procedure is usually carried out in patients who have been infertile for more than twelve or eighteen months— or sooner if the history suggests that disease is present in the pelvis.

Another significant cause of infertility in women is a disturbance of the female reproductive hormones. As already mentioned, ovulation depends on the interplay of hormones from the ovaries and the pituitary gland. If the pituitary gland is producing inadequate or excessive amounts of the relevant hormones, or the ovaries are not responding appropriately, fertility will be affected.

By measuring Follicle Stimulating Hormone and Luteinizing Hormone from the pituitary and Estrogen and Progesterone from the ovaries, hormonal status can be ascertained. If the levels of these hormones are upset, the result may be failure to ovulate or failure to maintain an early pregnancy. The measurement of these hormones at different stages of the menstrual cycle makes possible the determination of whether or not the hormonal system is functioning effectively.

The rise in Progesterone in the second half of the cycle is particularly important in diagnosis because this indicates whether the egg has left the ovary and whether the cells remaining in the ovary are producing sufficient Progesterone to sustain a pregnancy.

Prolactin is another hormone that may be important in infertility. This pituitary hormone is responsible for stimulating breast-milk production and, if present in excessive amounts in a nonpregnant woman, may result in infertility by blocking ovulation. Drugs, breast suckling, chronic anxiety, and pituitary disease may cause excess Prolactin.

In most women producing excess Prolactin, menstrual cycles may stop or be long and irregular, and milk may be secreted from the breasts. This type of infertility is akin to that occurring naturally when a mother breast-feeds a baby. Several measurements of Prolactin are necessary before a diagnosis of a Prolactin-associated disorder can be considered reliable, because anxiety can significantly affect the level of this hormone.

Infertility can also result from removal of the Fallopian tubes following an ectopic pregnancy or from endometriosis, which occurs when the tissue that lines the uterus (the endometrium) grows on various organs in the pelvis. The most usual sites of migration of endometrial tissue are the surface of the ovaries, behind the uterus, and within the Fallopian tubes.

Endometriosis is suspected if a woman in her twenties or thirties develops pain at ovulation or before or during her periods or experiences uncomfortable intercourse. However, many women with endometriosis have no symptoms except for infertility.

Endometriosis can occur as small spots, lumps, or cysts in the pelvis, and it causes infertility by preventing passage of eggs from the ovaries to the tubes, by blocking the pathway of sperm cells or eggs within the tubes, or by some as yet uncertain mechanism involving the production of chemicals that inhibit tube function or fertilization. The diagnosis is usually made from history and by visual inspection of the pelvis by means of laparoscopy.

Women with fibroids—round growths in the uterus—may also be infertile. These growths are not cancerous, but they may cause heavy or painful periods. Sometimes they cause infertility by blocking the tubes or growing into the lining of the uterus, or they may impair implantation, resulting in early abortion.

Fibroids may be indicated by the history and physical examination and confirmed by laparoscopy and curetting of the uterus.

Sometimes fibroids do not affect fertility, and it may be difficult for the doctor to decide whether this is the case. This difficulty may result in hesitancy on the doctor's part to offer treatment that requires major surgery and that may not overcome the infertility problem.

Adhesions are bands of fibrous tissue in the pelvis that may develop after infection or surgery. They are a very common cause of infertility and may produce the problem by preventing release of the egg from the ovary or impeding the passage of the egg to, or within, the tube. They may also cause pain with ovulation or intercourse and thereby reduce sexual activity. They are diagnosed by laparoscopy.

A damaged cervix may cause infertility, either because of an inability to produce the mucus that aids sperm transport or by being mechanically "incompetent" and thus unable to provide enough support for a pregnancy to continue beyond twelve weeks.

Are there other causes of infertility to which both partners may contribute?

Incompatibility between male sperm cells and the female genital tract may be a cause of infertility. Normally one of the functions of the female genital tract is to activate sperm cells, which, on contact with the fertile-type mucus produced by the cervix, are recharged, swimming more vigorously and consuming more energy. Incompatibility between sperm and mucus can be the result of antibodies present in the cervix, infection in the cervix, or the absence of mucus that promotes sperm movement at the time of ovulation.

An antibody is a protein produced by the body's immune (defense) system in response to an intruder, and one of its functions is to render intruders harmless. Antibody production is provoked by antigens, which are proteins that serve to identify intruders in the body.

The presence of sperm antibodies is diagnosed by means of a blood or cervical mucus test involving both partners. Male or female partners may produce antibodies to sperm cells. The antibodies fix on antigens that are on the surface of sperm cells, and as a result the sperm cells may no longer function effectively. For example, sperm cells immobilized by antibodies in the cervical mucus will not be able to penetrate the mucus to gain access to the uterus and Fallopian tubes.

Such problems of sperm-mucus incompatibility may be difficult to diagnose because this inactivation is quite normal during all except the fertile phase of the cycle. Thus, in diagnosing this problem, the sperm cells must be deposited at the cervix close to the time of ovulation and then their activity assessed. The test for diagnosing this type of abnormality is the "post-coital" (Huhner's) test. The mucus is collected from the cervix several hours after intercourse and studied under the microscope to examine the result of the sperm-mucus interaction.

More information may be gained by testing both the husband's and a donor's sperm cells with both the wife's and a donor's cervical mucus (Kremer test).

What is idiopathic infertility?

Idiopathic infertility is the term used to describe the situation in which there is no apparent cause of infertility.

The diagnosis follows a thorough assessment that fails to indicate a cause of the problem. In about 10 percent of couples with a infertility problem, the unsatisfactory diagnosis of idiopathic infertility is all that can be achieved with the present state of knowledge. However, such couples may become pregnant without any treatment: 40 percent after two years' infertility. Or they may become pregnant with the help of the test-tube-baby method.

Can psychological factors affect fertility?

Yes, this is apparent from examples of women in acute stress situations who stop ovulating and menstruating.

Anxiety about fertility can itself have profound effects as in the following examples.

- A woman may so desperately want to have a child that she comes to believe that she is pregnant; periods may stop and she may even begin producing milk. The hormonal upheaval involved in this situation means that the pregnancy that is so greatly desired becomes an impossibility because it has caused ovulation to stop.
- A woman who consciously pursues treatment for infertility may have such strong subconscious forces that she avoids intercourse during the fertile part of the cycle. The subconscious factors may be related to hostility toward her husband, fear of pregnancy or death during childbirth, or ambivalence about becoming pregnant.

There may be other ways not as yet well understood in which psychological factors influence fertility. Generally, however, most psychological disturbances in couples with infertility problems arise from—rather than cause—the infertility.

What treatments are available for infertility?

The treatment depends on the diagnosis.

In men, if sperm production is the problem, a detailed understanding of the cause of this is necessary before appropriate treatment can be given.

In some men, male hormones such as Testosterone may overcome a deficiency. Clomiphene (trade name, Clomid), a fertility pill first used in women, may also help stimulate sperm production. The drug Bromocriptine may cure infertility due to high levels of Prolactin hormone, a rare cause of infertility in the male.

27

If impaired fertility is due to an infection in the male genital tract such as in the prostate gland or testes, antibiotics are given. These may clear blockages of the system or, alternatively, enable sperm production. General anti-inflammatory drugs, such as anti-prostaglandins, may prove helpful also.

Men who have sexual problems associated with depression may be helped by anti-depressant drugs. However, these drugs may have side effects that reduce potency. Generally, drugs are helpful in at most 20 to 25 percent of male infertility problems.

Another treatment that may be considered is the surgical correction of varicoceles (varicose veins of the testes), but such treatment has a very low success rate.

Because many of the treatments for male infertility are relatively ineffective, men with problems of sperm production may be offered artificial insemination by donor (AID). Although this method of conception is less than ideal, it does give couples wishing to have a family an opportunity to use the wife's genetic material, and a situation in which the husband's physical characteristics (such as body build, eye color, complexion, height, hair color) can be matched with those of the donor of the sperm cells.

Another advantage of AID is that it has a much higher success rate than treating male infertility problems in other ways. About 65 percent of couples achieve a pregnancy within six months of starting AID treatment, and 80 percent do so within twelve months. These pregnancy rates are similar to those occurring in normally fertile couples.

Men with problems such as impotence (inability to achieve penile erection) or difficulty in ejaculating require different treatment. These problems may be related to early-childhood or adolescent experiences associated with sexuality, anxiety about expressing sexual feelings, or marital difficulties. If the GP, gynecologist, or infertility specialist cannot help, then it may be worthwhile consulting a sexual counselor, such as a psychiatrist, a clinical psychologist, or a gynecologist with specific training in treating these disorders. The resolution of psychological problems associated with infertility is very important, as treatment of physical disorders may result in a pregnancy, but persistent sexual problems may eventually disrupt the marriage.

Once again, in women, the treatment is determined by the diagnosis.

In the past, tubal disease has been treated either by flushing the tubes or by surgery.

The tubes may be flushed in the doctor's office with a gas. This is called the Ruben's test. The gas may be heard passing through the tubes, or the woman may feel pain in the shoulder—this is "referred" pain from the diaphragm resulting from the passage of gas from the Fallopian tubes. A more thorough method of flushing the tubes is with fluid. Flushing, however, is not very effective in treating tubal infertility, as only minor blockages can be removed.

Surgery is frequently advised when the tubes are blocked. The overall pregnancy rate following surgery on the tubes is only about 30 percent, or 40 percent if microsurgery is used, but in certain types of tubal repair, such as reversal of clip sterilization, the success rate may be much higher, whereas when tubal disease is severe the success rate is considerably lower—10 to 20 percent.

In reversal operations, the portion of the tube damaged by sterilization is cut out and the ends are rejoined. In general, the success rate of reversal depends on the length of healthy tube remaining. If only a few millimeters of tube have been damaged by the placement of a clip, then the success rate may be as high as 80 percent, but if more than half of the tube has been damaged by the sterilization procedure, the success rate of reversal varies from 10 to 40 percent.

Sometimes the blockage in the tube is at the outer end, where the fimbriae—the fingerlike fronds nearest the ovary—are stuck together by adhesions. Using microsurgery, adhesions can be dissected away, thus allowing a passage through which the eggs can enter the tube.

Fibroids of the uterus that require treatment can be removed by surgery. The growths are cut out of the uterus, and the uterine wall is rejoined.

If endometriosis is responsible for infertility, drug therapy, either alone or in combination with surgery, is available.

When the disease is mild, use of the drug Danocrine (trade name, Danazol) or Progestogens (Progesterone-like drugs) may be sufficient to cure it, but if the endometriosis has caused large cysts or nodules, particularly if this has affected the ovaries, surgery—as well as drug treatment—is usually required.

Sometimes it is quite clear that drug therapy will not cure the endometriosis, and in such cases Danocrine is given before surgery to make the operation safer and more effective. Drugs such as Danocrine act by reducing the production and blocking the action of the female hormone Estrogen, thus reducing growth of endometrial tissue, which is the basic component of the disease process.

Treatment of endometriosis is a complicated affair and considerable explanation, supervision, and counseling is required in order that the best result is obtained in the shortest possible time, and also so that any recurrence of endometriosis is recognized at an early stage.

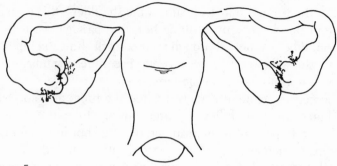

Figure 5.
Tubes blocked at outer end, preventing eggs from passing from ovary to the tube.

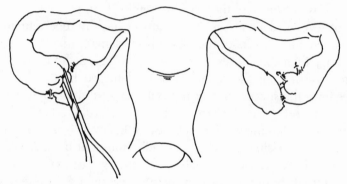

Outer end of the tube opened (left) with fine scissors, aided by microscope.

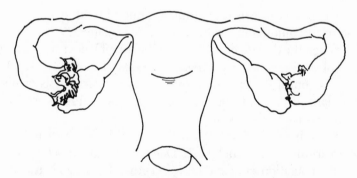

Left tube now open; procedure will be repeated on right tube. This operation often fails; IVF and ET may be needed.

The treatment of hormonal causes of infertility requires identification of the hormone abnormality, the most common treatment for which involves the use of fertility pills.

If ovulation is not occurring, Clomiphene is often used. This

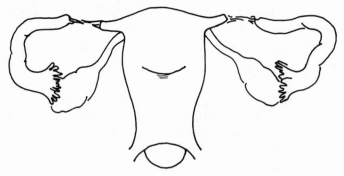

Figure 6.
Sterilization: destruction of inner one-fourth of tubes.

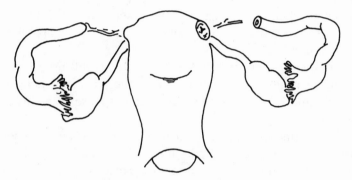

Reversal of sterilization: ends of tube (right) trimmed, ready to be rejoined.

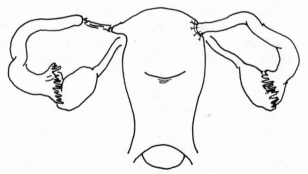

Tube rejoined by microsurgery: this operation has a good success rate. Left-tube reversal is carried out in the same manner.

drug stimulates the release of Follicle Stimulating Hormone (FSH) and Luteinizing Hormone (LH) and is given usually from the fifth to the ninth day of the menstrual cycle. The dosage, which varies from one to four tablets daily, is calculated on the basis of whether ovulation returns, as determined by temperature or mucus charting, or blood measurements of the hormone Progesterone.

If Clomiphene does not produce the desired response, pituitary hormones such as Human Chorionic Gonadotrophin or human pituitary extracts of the same hormones may be given. These substitute for FSH and LH.

If the infertility problem is caused by excess production of the hormone Prolactin, the drug Bromocryptine (trade name, Parlodel) may be given. This is used every day, and the dose is increased gradually until the level of Prolactin is reduced to normal.

Ovulation, menstruation, and pregnancy often follow the use of fertility drugs, but they may have some side effects. If the ovaries are overstimulated, pain may occur or cysts may form in the ovaries. If pain occurs when these drugs are being taken, use of the drugs should be discontinued and a doctor consulted. Cysts usually disappear without other treatment.

Another problem arises if the dose of the fertility drug is too great, resulting in multiple pregnancies—with the attendant increased risk to mother and fetuses. For this reason the response to the drugs must be monitored very carefully.

New hormone preparations are improving the treatment of hormone disorders. For example, a chemical substance that triggers the release of the pituitary hormones—commonly called a releasing factor—is available and in limited use.

Antibiotics may cure the problem if incompatibility between the sperm and the cervical mucus is due to infection, but treatment is more difficult if antibody formation immobilizes sperm cells. Intrauterine insemination with a partner's sperm cells has been tried but may not be successful because the antibodies may be present also in uterine fluid.

Treatments previously recommended to overcome the problem of antibody formation involved several months of either sexual abstinence, or the use of a condom to eliminate contact between the semen and the vagina. The rationale was that antibody production would decline with the elimination of contact; but the results of these treatment methods have proved disappointing. Suppression of antibody response with drugs such as Cortisone has also met with little success.

At present, couples with antibody problems are being treated by *in vitro* fertilization because if the sperm cells can penetrate the egg in the laboratory, it may be possible to bypass the antibodies present in the female genital tract. Embryos have been grown successfully in such patients.

The procedures of *in vitro* fertilization and embryo transfer are making possible the promising form of treatment that is described in detail in the following chapters.

In couples with no obvious cause of infertility (idiopathic infertility), treatments are sometimes offered in the hope that they may overcome some unidentified factor causing the problem.

Clomiphene is often used for six months in an attempt to ensure that ovulation is occurring regularly, and that adequate hormone levels following ovulation are maintained to make certain that any embryo formed encounters a suitable uterine environment in which to grow and develop.

Bromocryptine has been used also when the cause of infertility is in doubt, but it is uncertain whether it is helpful to reduce normal levels of the Prolactin hormone to very low levels. In view of uncertainties about the precise role of Prolactin in conception, this treatment may be unwise.

It is important for couples with unknown causes of infertility to be aware that 40 percent will become pregnant in the third or fourth year of so-called infertility. And even after this time, pregnancy may still occur.

How does infertility affect couples emotionally?

Some of the normal responses to infertility experienced by couples have been well described by Concern, a West Australian group of infertile couples who have formed a self-help group for mutual support. Normal responses include:

1. *Surprise.* The first and most common response is one of surprise. The couple feel surprised that pregnancy is not occurring. They also feel surprised that other couples find it easy to become pregnant, when they have been trying for a much longer period of time without success.

2. *Denial.* Couples may deny that there is a problem with their inability to conceive. This obviously results in a delay in seeking help. Some may deny to their friends and family that they even want children.

3. *Isolation.* A partner may feel isolated within his or her own relationship with the other. Therefore, one partner may be ready for a family quite a while before the other. The couples may feel isolated in their search for investigations and treatments. The male ego may be a barrier for some couples being investigated as a couple.

The couple may feel isolated from the community and from their friends who are conceiving readily. Many community activities center around children. For the infertile couple, seeing so many family situations can be very painful. Couples may find it difficult to meet others in the neighborhood, especially if the wife is working. This can lead to social isolation because of the lack of common interests.

4. *Anger.* The anger may be justified or unjustified. It may be directed at the people around the couple, the family, friends, the doctor and hospital staff. Even in the best doctor–patient relationship, the couple feel helpless.

They feel angry because they are losing control of their life plans. Their lives become centered around investigations and treatments.

They feel angry because they have to wait for appointments and then for results. Quite often they sit in a doctor's waiting room full of pregnant women, with only literature on childbirth and childcare to read.

They feel angry because they have to be exposed to inconvenience, pain, and indignity, when others achieve pregnancy so easily. They feel angry at friends and acquaintances who are all too ready to give advice as to how to attain pregnancy and seemingly take their own children for granted. Some feel angry when others, who have children, envy their childless state.

They may feel angry because they have to listen to their own parents' expectations of being grandparents and their not understanding the infertile couple's plight and the need for such intensive investigation when they themselves had no trouble conceiving.

The anger may be directed at the other partner in the relationship. One may feel that the partner is not understanding enough of the situation and not providing enough emotional support. Women may feel this especially at the time of menstruation. One partner may be as concerned about their infertility as the other but is not prepared to continue investigation and treatment, even if these are necessary for conception or the possibility of conception.

Couples feel angry that their sexual relationships are interfered with to such an extent that they can no longer be spontaneous. Sexual intercourse is on demand, depending on the time of the month, the fall and rise of the woman's temperature, and the requirements of investigations.

The anger may be directed at themselves. Couples may feel angry because they feel that they cannot cope with the complexity of the problem and would like to seek help but feel concerned that there might be something psychologically wrong with them, as many people around them make them feel this way.

5. *Guilt and Unworthiness.* The couple may feel guilty because they have been taking contraceptives to avoid pregnancy until establishing themselves financially.

One of the partners may carry the guilt alone, because of a previous affair, infection, abortion, or adoption, the knowledge of which has not been shared with the other partner.

This guilt may lead to a bargaining situation. Individuals may go to extremes to prove to God that they are sorry so that He might grant them a baby. For instance, they might involve themselves in many voluntary research projects. Doctors may see couples exposing themselves to almost unrealistic treatments with a high risk of side effects in the hope that even if the treatment is not successful, God will see that they are genuine in their efforts.

One partner may feel unworthy because he or she cannot give the other partner a child. Partners may feel that they are not contributing to society by being parents—parenthood may appear to be a passport to acceptance as a respectable citizen. Children are seen by many to be credentials to adulthood. To some couples deprived of children, there seems to be nothing to work for.

6. *Depression.* Depression can be intense. The whole body feels battered, both physically and emotionally, and failure is an everyday occurrence. Everywhere there is visual evidence of reproduction, pregnancy, and parenting, even in nature. For the infertile couple, every month provides evidence of failure, and even if some strive to forget, their bodies won't let them.

Some situations can be particularly depressing: christenings, a birth announcement, watching friends having their third or fourth pregnancy. There is a feeling of desperation that life is passing them by and that they don't fit into the community.

7. *Grief.* The couple grieve because of a feeling that their reproductive systems have stopped functioning. They may feel that part of them is dying slowly.

They grieve at the inability to give a partner a child, their parents a grandchild; at their inability to experience pregnancy and childbirth; at their losing a life goal.

The grief is experienced every month, month after month, year after year. Partners become physically and emotionally exhausted.

There are times when the couple may believe that they have

finally achieved a pregnancy and they may look for the signs. Some women experience morning sickness, sore breasts, and extreme tiredness. Even when the period does arrive, they can believe for some time that they are experiencing a threatened miscarriage. Some couples take repeated urine samples for pregnancy testing, hoping for a positive result.

It is emotionally draining, especially for those who do not have regular monthly cycles and those who have no known cause of their infertility.

Because infertility is not a visible condition, couples grieve alone.

As a person can only tolerate so much pain, some couples reach a stage of acceptance. . . . They learn to accept the fact that they can't cope all that well, all of the time.

8. *Acceptance.* Couples learn to avoid painful situations and to tolerate painful remarks, or to avoid the person making them. They learn to adjust to a different lifestyle. When a couple reaches this stage, the relationship is usually very close.

The fact that some couples do come to a stage of acceptance does not mean that they have given up hope.

They continue to hope for a new treatment that will enable them to have a child, or for their turn to come up on an adoption waiting list.

These insights, published with the permission of Concern, indicate the ways in which infertility can touch the emotional life of each partner and confront a relationship with intense, and often unexpected, stresses.

Suddenly expectations may be shattered; family and friends may react strangely; feelings of resentment or guilt may surface during discussions between partners.

Responses to infertility range across a wide spectrum. Some couples reach a stage of acceptance quickly; others pass through the stages described over many years, during which they may try every possible treatment.

An Australian woman wrote in June 1982 of the destructive effect that infertility was having on her marriage:

I will be 39 in July and do not have much time in which to produce babies. The situation is affecting my marriage.

I gave myself to the end of this year to become pregnant (having tried to have a baby for the past five years), and I decided that if I wasn't, then I had best leave my husband and let him look for a younger, more productive lady to have babies with.

This will be a very sad thing, as Martin and I have everything going for us but children.

Talking with other couples who share problems of infertility, and with counselors, can often help. And working through difficulties with a partner can deepen and strengthen a relationship and make it possible to take positive steps toward resolving this life crisis.

What are the options aside from treating infertility?

Adoption is one alternative for couples wanting a child, and it involves a legal process that makes a child a full member of a new family. Once an adoption order is made by a court, the adoptive parents have the same rights and responsibilities with regard to the child as do biological parents. The adoptive parents commit themselves to a lifetime of caring for the child and of the responsibilities of parenthood.

At present, adoption is extremely difficult in many Western countries. There are many categories of couples who are not accepted as potential adoptive parents—on the basis of age, financial status, marital stability, and general health. These restrictions are extremely stringent and have been made tougher because of the small number of children available. It is uncertain also whether the barriers to adoption are realistic in terms of choosing the most suitable couples.

Even if the couple is fortunate enough to be able to adopt, the waiting time can be from three to eight years.

Intercountry adoption is possible but not necessarily an easier or quicker way to obtain a child. Many of the systems developed are clumsy and expensive, and sometimes an adoption attempt results in great disappointment. In addition, many couples are sensitive to the possible problems of rearing a child of another nationality.

It is the decline in the number of children available for adoption that will probably lead to a system of surrogate (caretaker) pregnancies (see Chapter 10).

Fostering children suits some couples who have adjusted to roles other than parenthood in relation to children, but many couples find it difficult to rear, look after, and learn to love a child who soon leaves the home.

Other couples do not pursue adoption or fostering but retain contact with children through participation in activities involving the care of young children, such as Boy Scouts and Girl Scouts.

Teaching is another occupation that brings adults into close contact with children, albeit in tightly defined circumstances.

Couples who come to terms with regret about not being able to have children often find new energy and interest and pursue rewarding occupations, hobbies, and leisure activities. There is no doubt that some couples without children enjoy happier marriages than those who find difficulty in coping with the stresses of parenthood.

Occasionally, couples who cannot have children seek to dissolve their marriage. Although dissolution of the marriage in these circumstances may result in considerable unhappiness, the resentment sometimes evident as a result of infertility suggests that dissolution and subsequent remarriage may be preferable in the long term.

3

Development of the
Test-Tube-Baby Program

Scientists and doctors involved in the "test-tube-baby procedure" have developed the necessary techniques in response to the lack, or relatively low success rate, of other options. In the late 1960s, when the techniques were being developed for use in humans, the desperation of many patients with infertility problems was becoming particularly acute. This was due to two main factors.

First, the number of children available for adoption started to decline markedly. The main reasons for this were the ready availability of therapeutic abortion and the increasing support for single mothers wishing to keep a child.

The second factor was a recognition that the surgical treatment of tubal surgery did not restore the tubes in many women.

As mentioned previously, surgery to repair damaged Fallopian tubes has an overall success rate of only about 30 percent. The basic reason for this is that surgery is a relatively indelicate procedure for restoring the fine mechanisms of the tube.

The work that can be done by the surgeon is limited to unblocking the tube, either by excising a small portion or by removing adhesions. Very often, however, the problem extends beyond a simple blockage. The muscle that forms the main substance of the tube and the delicate cilia that move back and forth to provide currents for egg and embryo transport may be damaged. And although surgeons can remove a blockage, they cannot restore these other crucial functions of the tube.

Microsurgery performed under high magnification aroused hope as a means of improving the results of tubal surgery. Undoubtedly microsurgery has enabled greater success with tubal repairs because more gentle and accurate surgery is possible, but although the success rate has improved somewhat, tubal surgery is still frequently unsuccessful.

In view of the promise of microsurgery and with access to more experienced surgeons, many couples sought second and third repair operations on the tubes.

Numerous other approaches to improving treatment of tubal infertility have been attempted.

Earlier this century, when the tubes were severely damaged, surgeons experimented with placing the ovary in the uterus, hoping that fertilization and embryo growth would occur once the egg was in the uterine cavity.

Although a small number of pregnancies did result from this procedure, it involved considerable danger. In the first place, the transferred ovary could become diseased, necessitating its removal. Second, if pregnancy did occur, the uterus was in danger of rupturing along the scar formed to facilitate the transfer of the ovary. A low success rate, combined with such hazards, led to a general abandonment of this approach.

As more becomes known about ovulation and fertilization, it may be possible to improve or modify the procedure in some way. It has been established that human embryos fertilized in the uterus will develop and grow there, and pregnancies have been achieved recently using this procedure.

Another alternative to repairing damaged tubes is to transplant a tube from a donor. This has been achieved in some animal species, and microsurgery makes it an increasingly promising prospect in humans. Such a transplant requires that muscle tissue from the donor tube be joined to the recipient's uterus and that the blood vessels be reconnected skillfully.

Although these procedures are technically feasible, the drugs used to suppress rejection of transplanted tissues are very toxic, and most doctors will consent to their use only when life is threatened.

Tubal transplants may provide a practical alternative if improvements occur in microsurgical techniques, less toxic drugs are available to suppress rejection of the transplant, and the matching of donors and recipients becomes more accurate, thus minimizing the risk of rejection.

The possibility of replacing damaged tubes with artificial tubes has also been considered.

Such a procedure was carried out on one patient at the Queen Victoria Medical Centre in Australia in 1969 and led indirectly to the beginning of the test-tube-baby program in Melbourne. A plastic capsule was devised to enable the sperm and the egg to meet outside the ovary, and in the event of an embryo's forming, the artificial system was designed to enable delivery of the embryo to the uterus. The attempt was technically successful, but infection occurred in the artificial tube and eventually necessitated its removal.

In 1969, after members of the Queen Victoria Medical Centre presented a report on the artificial tube operation at a national conference, Dr. Neil Moore of Sydney University, a reproductive biologist working in animal research at Jerilderie in the state of New South Wales, suggested the possibility of egg collection, laboratory fertilization, and transfer of the early embryo to the patient to overcome tubal infertility.

Members of our program visited Jerilderie, and it was clear that both laboratory development of embryos from eggs that had been fertilized in the sheep as well as embryo transfer were technically feasible, although problems remained. At that stage, IVF had not been accomplished in the sheep, although in mice the laboratory fertilization of eggs and sperm cells had been achieved and embryo transfers and pregnancies had followed.

A few years later, Dr. Bob Edwards, working at Cambridge University in the late 1960s, started collecting human eggs which he attempted to fertilize in the laboratory, Dr. Edwards was able to achieve apparently normal embryo growth to the eight- and sixteen-cell stage.

In Melbourne, interest in the work of Dr. Edwards among clinicians and researchers at both the Queen Victoria Medical Centre (affiliated with Monash University, and where the clinical infertility work was headed by Dr. John Leeton) and at the Royal Women's Hospital (affiliated with the University of Melbourne, and where the Reproductive Biology Unit was headed by Ian Johnston) led to the formation of a collaborative team. This joint approach developed despite a number of unsuccessful attempts to devise other methods to overcome tubal infertility that had contributed to a general feeling of pessimism. Members of the team agreed that the project, even if it did not overcome the immediate problem of infertility, might lead to advances in the area of contraceptive development or in the understanding of abnormal embryo development. Perhaps the work would help fill some of the large gaps evident in knowledge about human eggs and sperm cells, the fertilization process, and the development of embryos. The main motivating factor was to develop an improved method of treating tubal infertility, as this would be of potential benefit to a substantial group of patients.

Gradually, outstanding research workers were recruited to the project. Among them was Dr. Alex Lopata, a senior lecturer in the Monash University Department of Obstetrics and Gynaecology, who joined the research team in 1970. His visits to Germany, the United

States, and England had convinced him of the potential of *in vitro* fertilization.

Meanwhile, Dr. Bob Edwards at Cambridge joined Dr. Patrick Steptoe at Oldham but although they published their techniques in some detail they failed to obtain any successful pregnancies. The Melbourne collaborative team was assisted by Dr. Moore, Dr. R. Lawson of Werribee Research Institute (near Melbourne), and other visiting reproductive biologists.

In Melbourne a small discussion group of leading reproductive scientists was formed that included Drs. Bryan Hudson, Henry Burger, David de Kretser, and Jim Brown. This group met regularly to review the IVF research and to make suggestions.

From 1970 to 1972 the Melbourne team collected eggs when operating on ovaries and also when using the technique of laparoscopy, which was developed by Dr. Patrick Steptoe in England. Dr. Lopata examined the eggs and devised his own criteria for assessing their ripeness and growth—information essential in developing the procedure.

By 1973 the Melbourne work was sufficiently advanced for an attempt at IVF and ET. To the delight of all concerned, two patients at the Queen Victoria Medical Centre appeared to achieve early pregnancies on the basis of evidence from hormone (chemical) tests. Although neither pregnancy continued beyond a few days, the objective of bypassing tubal blockage seemed to be close at hand, because success had come so rapidly. However, it would be another seven years before a baby was born in Melbourne with the help of IVF and ET.

Reviewing these frustrating years, we find that our research methods are open to criticism. Although we were content to obtain limited success in fertilization and embryo growth, we know now that unless embryos from the vast majority of couples can be grown in the laboratory, it is unlikely that the system is working well enough for pregnancies to occur. In other words, we set our goals too low. A better approach would have been to investigate more systematically methods of collecting mature eggs and growing and fertilizing them in culture.

At one point, despondency about the technique persuaded the team to try for fertilization of a human egg and sperm cell, and embryo growth, in sheep. After collecting a mature egg from a patient, we placed it and sperm cells from her husband in the sheep oviduct (the animal equivalent of the Fallopian tube.) But although the sperm cells survived in this environment, we were unable to find any trace of the egg. In some ways we were relieved at the failure of this experiment as it may have been difficult to convince the community that a sheep was an appropriate place for human fertilization and early embryo development.

By 1978 embryo formation was being achieved in 10 to 20 percent of patients, but pregnancies still eluded us.

It was at this time that Drs. Edwards and Steptoe announced the birth of Louise Brown in England, and, although disappointed at not having succeeded first, we were pleased to have confirmation of the possibilities of the technique.

Another significant event in our eventual success occurred in 1979, when a young reproductive physiologist, Alan Trounson, who had worked with Dr. Moore at Jerilderie, and later at Cambridge, in the area of freezing and thawing cattle embryos, joined the IVF team.

Dr. Trounson has since made several important contributions to our technique. He devised a quality control system for the culture fluids that entailed preliminary testing of mouse eggs and embryos: If the fluid would support the development of animal material, it was more likely to be suitable for the precious human eggs and embryos. At this time, the English team members had no such quality control system, but they and many other teams around the world have since included preliminary testing in their work.

By the end of 1979 success seemed imminent: many embryos were growing apparently normally in the tissue culture system. Then, a patient at the Royal Women's Hospital became pregnant.

Shortly after the birth of Candice Reed—the first "test-tube baby" success in Australia—the teams at the Queen Victoria Medical Centre and the Royal Women's Hospital decided to go their separate ways. This meant that the two research scientists, Drs. Lopata and Trounson, no longer worked together. Dr. Lopata went to the Royal Women's Hospital, and Dr. Trounson stayed at the Queen Victoria.

This enabled Dr. Trounson to exert more influence on the overall scientific direction of the Queen Victoria Medical Centre program. He was influential in the routine use of fertility pills to stimulate egg development, the quality control system for the cultural fluids, and improvements in egg-ripening techniques. These measures, together with refinements in egg pick-up and embryo transfer, resulted in a series of pregnancies at the Queen Victoria Medical Centre in 1980.

Initially, the system of egg pick-ups was not very satisfactory, and eggs were recovered from only 30 to 50 percent of patients using the technique of laparoscopy. So, Dr. Peter Renou, an obstetrician and gynecologist with considerable expertise in mechanical matters—particularly repairing cars—turned his attention to the problem. He devised a fine-gauge needle with an internal coat of teflon. This virtually eliminated the problem of eggs' and embryos' sticking to the fine tube and resulted in successful egg pick-ups in more than 80 percent of patients. Members of the team also devised special catheters to facilitate the safe and gentle transfer of the embryo.

The routine use of fertility pills during the test-tube-baby procedure was first introduced at the Queen Victoria. Previously, Dr. Edwards had abandoned the use of fertility drugs to stimulate ovulation at a predictable time, preferring to work with the natural menstrual cycle. His studies indicated that the use of fertility pills could disturb the production of hormones necessary for a successful pregnancy.

Problems of logistics, however, made it impossible to rely on the natural cycle, for ovulation can occur at any time, day or night, which necessitates access to an operating room with only six to twelve hours notice. Since the Queen Victoria Medical Centre is a busy teaching hospital in the heart of Melbourne, its operating rooms need to be available for emergencies around the clock. And unless rooms and beds are booked in advance, there is little hope of obtaining them when necessary.

For this reason, and because we were unconvinced by Dr. Edwards's findings and had access to expert advice from Dr. Jim Brown on hormone responses to induced ovulation, we persevered with the fertility pill. This approach seemed reasonable, since pregancy often follows the use of fertility pills by women who are not ovulating and therefore the use of such pills should be compatible with IVF. This was shown to be true and all early successes at the Queen Victoria Medical Centre followed use of fertility pills.

Another advantage of this approach was that two or more eggs usually ripened in the ovaries instead of only one. This improved the chance of picking up several ripe eggs and consequently increased the likelihood of producing one or more embryos for transfer.

Subsequently we have found that the likelihood of pregnancy is greater for the transfer of three embryos (40 percent) than for two embryos (28 percent), which again is greater than for one (12 percent).

Several other discoveries proved to be important.

For some years it was thought that ripening of an immature egg in the laboratory was an impossibility. We discovered that by leaving eggs for five or six hours in the culture fluid prior to the addition of sperm cells, embryo growth was enhanced. Using a high-powered electron microscope, Dr. Henry Sathananthan of the Lincoln Institute in Melbourne was able to provide evidence of what seemed to be occurring. He was able to demonstrate physical differences, indicating greater maturity, in eggs left alone in the culture fluid for six hours, in comparison with those examined immediately after pick-up.

Previous attempts at fertilization of immature eggs demonstrated a high rate of failed or incomplete fertilization. Consequently, maturing eggs for four to six hours before the addition of sperm cells has become a routine practice and has resulted in a significantly increased success rate in embryo formation.

Similar work by Dr. Edwards has confirmed this finding, and occasionally he has left eggs for up to eighteen hours before adding sperm cells.

Originally, the culture fluid used for growing the eggs and embryos was extremely complex, containing more than 180 different substances. This "broth" contained most of the constituents of the serum portion of human blood and had been used for many years to culture animal eggs and embryos. The disadvantage of working with such a highly complex fluid is that it is unclear which of the ingredients are essential for success and which are unnecessary extras. Thus in the situation where the fluid fails to promote growth it is very difficult to pinpoint the chemical error or errors responsible.

We found with considerable relief that fertilization and normal embryo growth were possible when using much more simple culture fluids that contained only ten to twenty different substances and could be prepared in our own laboratory. By removing nonessential substances from the culture fluids, we gained valuable insights into the vital ingredients for egg and embryo growth and into the building blocks of early life. One thing is certain: It is very easy for toxic chemicals to gain access to the culture fluid and inhibit growth. Despite thorough washing and cleaning of laboratory apparatus, substances can pass into the fluid from glass and plastic tubes.

As the program has developed, many changes have been necessary because the system still works less effectively at some times than at others. Until the reasons for successes and failures are more clearly understood, a consistently high rate of success will remain elusive.

One change that became necessary during 1980 and 1981 had more to do with logistics than techniques. The clinical work of the program was transferred to St. Andrew's Hospital at the edge of Melbourne's central business district. This was because of demands for operating-room time and the necessity of ready access to hospital beds.

In 1982 this arrangement was replaced by a new Monash University Infertility Service at Epworth Hospital, also on the fringe of central Melbourne, which was established in order to increase the efficiency of treating the 2000 couples on the waiting list.

Meanwhile, the basic research continued at the Queen Victoria Medical Centre, and scientists from more than twenty countries visited Melbourne to learn the techniques involved. With pooling of knowledge from centers established by these scientists throughout the world, greater understanding of the critical factors in the success of the test-tube-baby method should develop rapidly.

Growing awareness of the value of the procedure in treating infertility was indicated in July 1982, when a workshop on how to establish an IVF clinic attracted forty-two doctors from eleven countries to Melbourne.

Currently, aside from making the program more reliable, a major aim is to develop embryo preservation using freeze–thaw procedures, because this will make the program more efficient. Another aim is the transfer of eggs from one woman to another, as this will enable women with absent or diseased ovaries to have children.

4

Whom Can the
Program Help?

The selection of suitable patients is an essential part of any *in vitro* fertilization clinic. It is not only disillusioning but even emotionally destructive for couples to undergo numerous unsuccessful treatment attempts only to discover that the chances of a pregnancy were minimal from the outset.

Conditions of infertility
that the treatment may overcome

The techniques of *in vitro* fertilization and embryo transfer were developed to enable conception in spite of blocked, damaged, or absent Fallopian tubes in those cases where the problem could not be solved by antibiotics or surgery.

The potential of these techniques is now recognized to be considerably greater, and the current success rate of the test-tube-baby procedure (see Chapter 8) is comparable to that of tubal surgery. In certain circumstances the IVF procedure is preferable to tubal surgery—for instance, when the tube is severely damaged at the outer end or along its length or if it is markedly shortened as a result of previous sterilization. Sometimes surgery to repair a tube is undertaken, but after its completion, adhesions and pain may occur and necessitate the removal of one or both Fallopian tubes.

There are other reasons for removal of tubes. An ectopic (tubal) pregnancy necessitates such action because of the danger of rupture of the tube and subsequent life-threatening complications. A damaged or previously infected tube may be the site of another infection. This calls for treatment for reasons other than the need to ease the discomfort.

47

An infected tube on one side of the pelvis may act as a focus for infection of a healthy tube on the other side. Because of this, a surgeon may recommend the removal of the severely infected tube.

If tubal surgery has been carried out but the operation has proved unsuccessful, some patients wonder about the feasibility of a second operation. Generally, the success rate of a second tubal repair is less than the first, but with the prospect of a more experienced surgeon and microsurgery, a second operation may make good sense.

When assessing a patient's suitability for a second tubal repair operation, the surgeon may suggest a laparoscopy, which, as described in Chapter 2, enables inspection of the ovaries and Fallopian tubes. At the same time, the surgeon can assess whether the alternative of *in vitro* fertilization and embryo transfer would be preferable.

If a woman is concerned that tubal surgery requires a major operation, involving several hours under anaesthetic and an incision ten to fifteen centimeters long in the lower abdomen, together with about a week in the hospital, she may prefer the test-tube-baby procedure as an alternative method of achieving a pregnancy, assuming that both techniques offer a comparable success rate.

Further surgery may also be required if a tubal repair operation is followed by a tubal pregnancy, which cannot succeed.

The cost is not very different and, except in carefully selected patients where tubal surgery is highly effective—such as after clip sterilization or when fine adhesions alone impair fertility—the success rate is comparable.

Despite thorough investigations, the cause of infertility cannot be identified in about 10 percent of couples, a situation described as *idiopathic infertility*.

This unsatisfactory diagnosis follows a comprehensive history-taking involving both partners, physical examinations, laparoscopy, tests to determine whether the Fallopian tubes are open, temperature charts, hormone assessments, and semen analyses.

The absence of abnormal findings in these tests, in association with regular intercourse for more than a year, constitutes idiopathic infertility. However, it is worth remembering that many couples in this situation still become pregnant—about 40 percent within the following two years. Because of the uncertainty of ever achieving a pregnancy, it seems reasonable for such couples to enter test-tube baby programs.

Originally, it was thought that *in vitro* fertilization might have a valuable role in helping to diagnose the problem in such couples; that is, failure of fertilization in the laboratory would indicate the presence of defects in the egg and/or sperm cells, undetectable by the usual tests. Our experience is that couples with no apparent cause of infertility develop embryos and become pregnant with nearly the same degree of success as couples with tubal disease. This indicates that in most couples with idiopathic infertility there is nothing wrong with either the sperm cells or the eggs. The cause of the infertility would seem to reside somewhere in the woman, but a means of determining the site of the problem has not yet been devised. Exposure of the egg to sperm cells in the laboratory makes it possible to bypass the unknown cause of infertility.

Because couples with idiopathic infertility may become pregnant without any treatment, it has been argued that they should not have the same priority in test-tube-baby programs as patients with, for example, tubal infertility. However, it is equally true that some patients with tubal infertility have a small chance of becoming pregnant, such as those with one open, but abnormal, tube.

The complexity of trying to organize waiting lists according to the severity of the infertility is so great that we have established a policy of giving all patients who have been infertile for one or more years the same priority on the waiting list, regardless of the cause.

Theoretically, the test-tube-baby program could provide an opportunity for men with low sperm counts to become fathers.

A sperm count of 20 million per milliliter of ejaculate is usually considered the cut-off point for fertility. Below this level, difficulties in conceiving are common.

The reason that so many sperm cells are required in the conventional system of conception is that the wastage of sperm cells is enormous. Of the millions of sperm cells that enter the vagina during intercourse, only about one hundred ever travel the length of a Fallopian tube. However, once they reach this region, the fertilization process is very efficient. Either the fluid in the Fallopian tubes or the sperm cells themselves help to break down the cells and gel-like coat that surrounds the egg, so that one sperm cell can eventually gain access.

When the *in vitro* fertilization technique was first attempted in humans, about 500,000 sperm cells were added to a single egg. This has since been reduced five- to ten-fold with complete success.

Even so, the addition of 50,000 to 100,000 sperm cells to the egg seems excessive when compared with the small number of sperm cells that reach the egg in the natural system. The reason for the larger number required in the laboratory situation is that they are thought to be needed to break down the outer coat of the egg because of the absence of factors normally produced by the tube that enable this to take place. Smaller numbers of sperm cells will be used to test this theory because, if fewer sperm are sufficient, this may have implications for the treatment of some types of male infertility.

Although 50,000 is still a relatively large number of sperm cells, it would seem a reasonable proposition that the test-tube-baby procedure could provide a possible means of overcoming the problem of a low sperm count—that is, less than 20 million.

One difficulty, however, is that low sperm counts are often accompanied by sperm cells of poor quality. Thus, men with counts below 20 million per milliliter of ejaculate tend to have motility (sperm movement) measurements that are also low. This poor motility reflects poor sperm structure and/or function. Thus 50,000 sperm cells from a man with a low sperm count are not equivalent to the same number from a man with a higher sperm count.

Despite this theoretical objection to using the test-tube procedure to help men with low sperm counts, experiments are under way on a small group with this problem. By mid-1982, one pregnancy had occurred where the male partner had a count of 12 million sperm per milliliter and a motility of 30 percent (normally, 70 percent or more sperm cells are motile). Also, embryos have been grown successfully using sperm cells from other men with counts between 10 and 20 million per milliliter, and motility between 30 and 70 percent. Most U.S. programs do not accept male-factor problems.

Another prospect for the future is to make the most effective use of a very few normal sperm cells by adding chemicals to dissolve the cells and coat surrounding the egg. By this means, it has been possible for scientists to show that one sperm cell can penetrate the egg in the laboratory.

When endometriosis is controlled by drugs or surgery, conception may occur in the conventional manner. However, tubal or ovarian damage or adhesions resulting from the disease may result in infertility, and *in vitro* fertilization is offered to such patients. Patients who do not become pregnant after AID (artificial insemination by donor sperm cells) are also offered this treatment.

Essential requirements for selection

Originally, women accepted for treatment had to be ovulating. However, now, if ovulation is not occurring naturally, fertility pills are given to ensure that ovulation can be stimulated before the women enter the program; women who do not ovulate naturally have become pregnant as a result of IVF.

It is important that the ovaries be accessible so that ripe eggs can be picked up during laparoscopy (see Chapter 5). A preliminary laparoscopy is carried out to ensure that this is so. If the ovaries are not accessible, an operation may clear away adhesions. If this is not possible or is unsuccessful, a patient may choose to accept donor eggs from another woman.

A normal uterus and a competent cervix are necessary so that pregnancy can proceed. The cervix also needs to be sufficiently open so that an embryo can be transferred into the uterus.

The male partner must be able to provide at least some normal, motile sperm cells. Semen samples are analyzed on three occasions. If any of the samples are abnormal, or if the male has difficulty producing a semen specimen at any point, then at the time of a satisfactory collection a portion of the semen is frozen. This substitutes for an unsatisfactory or failed semen sample taken after the egg pick-up.

Obese patients are asked to lose weight before being accepted, because obesity makes the egg pick-up procedure more difficult and less safe. Excess weight also interferes with the clarity of ultrasound pictures, which are used as an aid to determining the rate and stage of egg maturation. Weight reduction also has advantages if pregnancy occurs, because marked obesity is associated with a higher risk of complications during pregnancy.

Because fertility declines with increasing age, women over the age of forty are discouraged from joining the program. Although a pregnancy has occurred in a Melbourne woman over that age, the less-than-ideal success rate of the test-tube procedure, combined with declining fertility with increasing age, makes success less likely.

A small group of women who are forty or older has been included in the program to establish whether this age barrier is justified, for it is possible that *in vitro* fertilization and embryo transfer can overcome some of the disadvantages associated with aging in the natural system. If the decline in fertility with age is due to factors in the female reproductive system, then the program may be a suitable way to achieve pregnancy in older women.

A state of good general health is important if patients are to cope with pregnancy, birth, and child rearing. Well-recognized guidelines for maintaining an optimal standard of health include the following suggestions:

- avoid excess amounts of fatty or carbohydrate-containing foods
- exercise a moderate daily amount; if this is not possible, exercise for at least thirty minutes, three times a week
- sleep six to nine hours each night according to need
- stop smoking or reduce cigarette intake to a minimum; risks in pregnancy are reduced by smoking fewer than ten cigarettes a day
- reduce alcohol intake to a minimum during pregnancy
- prevent or control obesity
- make use of the immunization services offered by community health centers, particularly for rubella (German measles), which can cause fetal malformation if acquired during pregnancy
- stop any form of medication abuse; check with your doctor that any drugs taken routinely are not dangerous during pregnancy
- organize your occupation and leisure so that you learn how to relax.

During the treatment, there are times when relaxation is important. If you are the sort of person who finds this difficult, it may be helpful to join a relaxation class. These are run by clinical psychologists, yoga practitioners, behavioral therapists, general practitioners, psychiatrists, and physiotherapists. Not only will relaxation help in the various steps during each treatment attempt, but it is a great asset during pregnancy and childbirth.

Another factor taken into account in selecting patients for the program is stabilization of medical problems. If pelvic infection or endometriosis is present, the condition must be treated before a treatment attempt, because active disease may prevent the surgeon from gaining access to the ovaries for pick-up of eggs. Active disease in the pelvis may also interfere with pregnancy.

Couples with religious convictions should be sure before joining the program that these are compatible with all aspects of the treatment.

Psychological criteria

A realistic appreciation of the procedure is necessary because of the difficulties that may occur during treatment, and the likelihood that pregnancy will not result. Provided that couples fully understand the treatment, and feel up to meeting its demands, no further psychological criteria for selection are imposed.

Any infertility treatment imposes stress on the patient. The test-tube procedure makes its own particular demands (see Chapter 6), and couples need to be able to collaborate to a greater-than-usual degree with the medical and scientific team. Frequent visits to the hospital, a variety of diagnostic tests involving the taking of blood samples, the uncertainties of when admission to the hospital will occur and of whether eggs will mature appropriately, the doubts as to whether the laparoscopy will be successful, the further worry about whether fertilization and embryo growth will occur, and finally the anxiety of waiting to hear whether the embryo has been transferred successfully are—in combination—a formidable series of stresses.

In addition, it is discouraging to know that even if an embryo is transferred, only one in four will implant successfully. Although some patients are heartened that an embryo has developed in the laboratory, even if a pregnancy does not follow, others are deeply distressed and sometimes even guilt-ridden, as they may blame themselves for in some way contributing to the failure.

Until a couple has been involved in a treatment attempt, it is difficult to assess their ability to cope with the stresses involved. Thus the most reliable assessment of a couple's psychological suitability for the procedure can be made only after the first attempt. At this time, if one or both partners are very depressed or anxious about the treatment, they may be counseled to withdraw, temporarily or permanently, from the program.

In practice, very few couples wish to withdraw after one attempt, and the majority proceed to three or more attempts. Couples are often allowed as many treatments as they wish, although many unsuccessful couples give up after three or four tries. Some clinics allow as many attempts as a couple wishes; others limit to three to five attempts.

Other selection criteria

It makes no difference to the priority given to couples if they already have children—either adopted, conceived before the infertility problem occurred, or achieved through artificial insemination or a previous successful in vitro fertilization attempt. This policy has been criticized and may be changed. In the U.S., many programs give priority to couples with no children.

Most adoption agencies will not consider making a child available for adoption to a couple receiving treatment for infertility, but because of the very long waiting lists for the test-tube procedure and the uncertainty with regard to success, some agencies have made exceptions for couples who are on test-tube program waiting lists. Adoptions have gone ahead while test-tube treatment attempts are deferred, and patients treated in the program also include those who have succeeded already in adopting a child.

One good reason for attempting to adopt before joining a test-tube-baby program is that by the time a couple has been on a program waiting list and completed three or more treatments, the partners may be too old to be accepted as adoptive parents. Most agencies have a cut-off point for the age of both the husband and wife; it varies from thirty-five to forty-five years old.

The financial cost of the treatment may be a problem. Although the total cost of each treatment attempt, in late 1983, amounted to $3500 to $8000, most couples do not find cost a barrier. Being infertile, they usually have not had the expenses associated with rearing children and it is therefore often possible for them to save enough for several treatments. Financial aspects are less of a hindrance in Australia, where couples may take out a health insurance policy to cover most of the cost.

Another possible selection factor that has been considered is educational level or intelligence. The reason for reflecting on whether this should be considered during the selection process is the necessity for couples to understand the test-tube procedure and thus be in a position to give informed consent.

The consent form, signed before treatment by both partners, specifies that they understand the procedure, and in particular its risks; that it is uncertain whether fetal malformation may result from the procedure; that they accept the risks of laparoscopy; and that tests for fetal malformation will be offered during the pregnancy. There is no obligation for couples to have these tests or to act on the information obtained from such tests; any decision concerning a therapeutic abortion in the event of a malformation is the sole concern of the couple. Couples who do have a therapeutic abortion must postpone another attempt for two months.

The use of the consent form in medical procedures has limitations. It implies that patients are fully informed about the advantages and disadvantages of any procedure. However, the more complex the procedure, the more difficult it is to impart this information and to be certain that the patient understands all that has been discussed.

This is particularly true of *in vitro* fertilization and embryo transfer, as the reasons for success are still uncertain and the success rate may vary considerably from time to time even within the same clinic. These factors make it difficult to design a suitable consent form, or to assume that formal acceptance of the terms of such a form really amounts to fully informed consent. Nevertheless, it does imply a matter of good will between the therapist and the patient, ensures a measure of protection for the prospective parents, and provides a statement that an effort has been made to communicate as much as possible, given the current state of knowledge.

The information that team members try to impart includes an explanation of the procedures and a description of accompanying discomfort or pain; the extent of risks to the woman and the embryo (it is stressed that there may be unknown risks also); the availability of tests to detect fetal abnormality during the pregnancy (see pages 105–06); the likelihood of success; the source of any donated material used during the procedure; and discussion of other methods of infertility treatment and alternatives, such as adoption.

The relationship between partners is extremely important, for the treatment imposes stresses that can be handled more easily if mutual emotional support is given.

At a practical level, two heads are often found to be better than one. During interviews with members of the team, for example, the information is often understood better by one partner or the other. Each can ask questions about the treatment, and after the interview discussions will crystallize any differences between what partners understand will occur and why. Discrepancies can be resolved by contacting a member of the team.

Just as in the natural system of conception, both partners play an essential role, and it is preferable if prospective fathers attend interviews and are present during the embryo transfer. Their presence is essential at the time of egg collection.

Married couples are given selection preferences because of the great demand for IVF treatment, but since a supportive relationship is essential during treatment, it is probably best to postpone treatment if the marriage is in a period of instability.

5

The Treatment

One helpful way to describe the test-tube-baby procedure is to follow a couple—let us call them Diane and Michael—from start to finish of a treatment attempt.

Figure 20 (on page 79) shows the various stages of the treatment during the month of the egg pick-up and embryo transfer, and you may find it useful to refer to it while reading.

Entry into the program

Diane and Michael have been advised that a place has been set aside for them in the treatment program either this month or next.

The reason for imprecision in predicting exactly when treatment can start relates to the uncertainty associated with the commencement of menstrual periods, so a more than adequate pool of potential patients is notified about the possibility of treatment to ensure that the hospital quota for the month is filled. Preference is given to patients who have been waiting longer, and to those who failed the previous month because of unforeseen circumstances.

When Diane notices the start of her period, she telephones the infertility clinic: "My period began today. Can I start my *in vitro* treatment this month?"

She is asked to call back the next day for confirmation of acceptance for treatment, and she is also advised to take and chart her temperature each morning from now until she is told to stop.

"Yes," she is told the next day, "you're in. You need to see us and pick up your fertility tablets within the next three days."

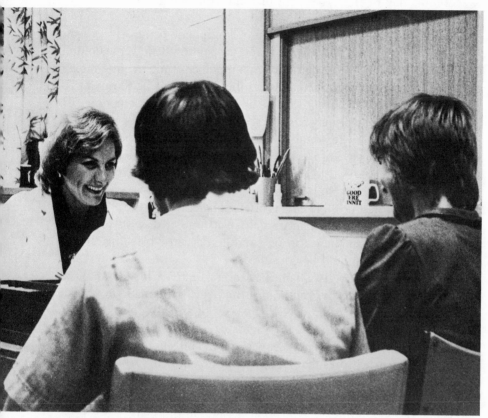

Figure 7. Preliminary interview: the male partner is involved in as many steps of the procedure as possible.

Fertility drugs

The main aim of the fertility drugs is to cause more than one egg to ripen, as this increases the chance that at least one healthy embryo will develop that can be transferred to achieve a pregnancy.

The use of fertility drugs also makes organization of the procedure considerably easier. Operating rooms can be pre-booked for egg pick-ups at times compatible with the staffing situation and other requirements of the hospital.

That afternoon, Diane sees the nurse who is organizing the treatment schedule, and at first visit she is given a prescription for the fertility drug Clomiphene (trade name, Clomid), which she collects from the hospital pharmacy. Clomiphene tablets are usually taken three times a day from the fifth to the ninth, or the second to the seventh, day of the cycle, the first day coinciding with the start of menstrual bleeding.

In a small number of patients, Clomiphene causes side effects, such as headache, rash, blurred vision, or pain in the lower abdomen. If any of these symptoms are severe, a member of the treatment team should be informed immediately, as the dosage may be too high.

If Clomiphene is not successful in stimulating egg ripening, the fertility drug Pergonal may be prescribed, either alone or in combination with Clomiphene. Pergonal is given by injection in various dosages during the early days of the cycle. Although it works differently from Clomiphene, the result is the same; that is, the development of several ripe eggs.

The greatest possible care is taken in determining the appropriate dosage of Pergonal. If the ovaries are overstimulated, cysts may form in the ovaries, and these can be painful and cause bleeding. If pain occurs, a doctor should be consulted.

Early in the cycle, Diane has several tests. A blood sample is obtained that enables hormone measurements to be made to provide a baseline for future reference. Vaginal swabs are taken also to ensure that there is no infection in the vagina or cervix. This is particularly important during embryo transfer because the infection may be carried into the uterus with resultant damage to the embryo.

If a serious infection is present, antibiotics are given, and treatment is deferred until the following month. If the infection is mild and has cleared up before the egg collection, treatment proceeds.

Estimating ovulation time

It is necessary to know accurately when ovulation will occur so that ripe eggs can be picked up just before they are released from the ovaries, and the rate at which the eggs are maturing is followed closely. Progress toward egg maturity is monitored by daily temperature measurements, Estrogen hormone levels, ultrasound and mucus scores, and, after admission to the hospital, by Luteinizing Hormone measurements. Previous menstrual cycle lengths are also taken into account.

The information about the rate of egg ripening determines when a woman enters the hospital for the egg pick-up and when an injection of another fertility drug, Human Chorionic Gonadotrophin (HCG), is given.

Temperature chart

Diane's daily temperature chart provides reassurance that ovulation has not occurred in the early days of the cycle and that she is not pregnant. The chart will be important after *in vitro* fertilization and embryo transfer in assessing whether a pregnancy has occurred and—if so—if it is continuing.

To take her temperature reliably, Diane has her chart, a thermometer, a pencil, and a clock beside her bed when going to sleep. She also checks that the mercury is below the 35°C (96°F) mark.

On waking, she takes her temperature before getting out of bed, talking, drinking, or eating. If the temperature is taken orally, the thermometer is kept under the tongue for four minutes; if taken vaginally, the thermometer remains in the vagina for three minutes.

Estrogen hormone level

The blood level of the hormone Estrogen is probably the most important of the measurements in predicting ovulation, for the level rises as the egg develops.

From Day 8, daily measurements are taken of this hormone in Diane's blood. (Had she been prescribed FSH in the form of Pergonal, these blood measurements would have commenced on Day 4.)

Experience with the treatment indicates that if the Estrogen level remains low, eggs are not developing adequately and pregnancy is not likely to occur. In this situation of a low Estrogen level, patients are advised to defer treatment for a month, or dosages of medications may be changed during the remainder of the cycle. In a later cycle, the dosage of the fertility drug may be increased or the type of drug changed, in a bid to produce a more effective stimulation of the ovaries.

Treatment may also be deferred if there is anything unusual about the menstrual cycle in the month before treatment, if a serious illness has occurred at this time, or if abnormal bleeding or pain occurs during the treatment cycle.

Ultrasound (sonar)

Another test carried out on about Day 7 and repeated closer to the day of ovulation is an ultrasonic scan of the ovaries. Ultrasound produces an image of body tissues—in this case, the ovaries.

During the scan a skilled technician moves a small device, from which sound-like waves are emitted, over the body surface. These sound waves penetrate the body and are reflected back according to the characteristics of a particular tissue. When the sound waves are directed toward the ovaries, an image of the fluid-filled follicles containing the developing eggs can be observed.

The size of the follicle indicates the degree of egg maturity. When the egg is immature, the follicle is only a few millimeters in size, but at full maturity it grows to about two centimeters. After the ripe egg leaves the ovary, the follicle collapses and fills with blood. It can be distinguished from the follicle by ultrasound.

Although ultrasound is very useful in determining the number and size of follicles, it is not 100 percent accurate, particularly in overweight patients or those with many adhesions or other physical abnormalities in the pelvis.

Diane is advised to have a full bladder for the ultrasound, so she experiments in advance to see how much fluid is needed in order to produce a feeling of fullness without pain.

Viewing a screen placed beside her during the second ultrasound, she can see several follicles. If no follicles are evident at this stage, consideration is given to abandoning the treatment for that month.

Mucus scores

Mucus produced by the cervix is also a useful indicator of the approach of ovulation.

In a simple, inexpensive test, mucus is taken at the time of speculum examination of the cervix and assessed according to amount, texture, and appearance.

A woman may keep her own daily chart of mucus characteristics as another guide to ovulation. The mucus characteristics reflect the level of Estrogen hormone, and they are assigned a score. When the score reaches a maximum, Estrogen is nearing its peak, and ovulation can be expected within the next day or two.

In the hospital

As a result of the information gained from the various tests described, Diane is admitted to the hospital on Day 11 of her cycle. Some patients are admitted earlier if the follicles are growing quickly as determined by Estrogen levels or ultrasound scans.

The main purpose of hospital admission is to enable more frequent tests to be carried out, and thus to obtain a more accurate determination of the rate of egg ripening. (This is achieved in most U.S. programs by outpatient attendance.) The date of admission usually allows sufficient time for doctors to intervene in the stimulated cycle by giving HCG to trigger the final stages of egg ripening.

Once checked in, Diane finds that she is relatively free to come and go as she pleases, as long as she tells the staff of her movements and provided that these do not interfere with urine collections and other tests. Within these limitations she is able to go out for a meal, to the movies, or for a walk. Relaxation during this time of waiting is extremely important.

Luteinizing Hormone level

A surge of Luteinizing Hormone (LH) indicates that the final development of the egg is under way, and it occurs after Estrogen reaches a high level.

The production of LH is monitored regularly and frequently in the urine. (Other clinics may measure LH by repeated blood tests.)

Once monitoring starts, Diane passes urine every three hours into the bottles provided, except at night when the collections are taken at midnight and 6 A.M.

Only a small amount of urine is desirable at each collection because if the urine is too dilute, the LH measurement is less accurate. The ability to provide a small volume of urine every few hours depends largely on the daily food and fluid intake. Diane finds that by restricting her drinks to four or five cups a day, she is able to adjust to the requirements.

In Diane's case, it is possible for the team to intervene in the control of the cycle before the LH surge starts. This intervention enables the egg pick-up to be performed during daylight or evening hours when staff and operating rooms are more likely to be available.

Diane is given an injection of HCG when the Estrogen reaches a critical level, and the egg pick-up is scheduled for thirty-two hours later.

If the LH surge starts before the HCG injection is given (this can easily happen because of the considerable individual differences between

61

the level of Estrogen at which the LH surge commences), egg pick-up is timed for twenty-six hours after the LH begins to rise. Recently the pregnancy rate has been higher in women whose eggs have been picked up after the natural LH rise, so unless there is a very good reason for giving the HCG injection, the spontaneous LH rise is preferred.

The timing of the pick-up procedure is very important because if the eggs are too immature, fertilization will not occur or, if it does, embryo development may be abnormal.

However, eggs' being a few hours short of full maturity does not seem to matter. Eggs kept in culture fluid for several hours do mature, and changes occur in the substance of the egg that allow normal fertilization. Also, eggs allowed to ripen in the laboratory for a few hours develop the ability to prevent more than one sperm cell from entering the egg.

Tests to determine the ripening rate of eggs are improving constantly. If it becomes possible to predict ovulation with greater precision, it is likely that the egg pick-up rate will increase from its present level of 80 to 90 percent, and the quality of the eggs may also improve. These factors could well increase the overall success rate of the treatment.

Currently, eggs remain in culture for five to twelve hours before sperm cells are added. But this is only an estimate, as some eggs may already be fully mature, and others may require a longer time to mature before the sperm cells are added.

Further detailed studies of eggs may help to determine the exact time each egg requires to ripen.

Another possible aid in the assessment of the appropriate time for the egg pick-up is the measurement of the hormone Progesterone. This hormone is produced just before ovulation and reflects the action of LH on the ovaries.

In the days before the pick-up procedure, Diane learns a great deal more about the treatment schedule as she talks to other women waiting in the hospital for their egg pick-ups or embryo transfers. There is a close feeling between these women, a sharing of hopes and disappointments. Some women who have become extremely well informed about the procedures now work as assistant therapists. They help the team by checking the collection times of urine and blood samples, the availability of hormone level results, the injection times for HCG, and the subsequent egg pick-up times. Other interested patients assist in the overall organization of the program.

As the main purpose of hospital admission is to allow closer scrutiny of hormone levels as an indication of egg maturity, it may be possible in the future to organize accommodation that is more like a motel than a hospital. This would reduce the cost and provide less formal surroundings during the difficult waiting period.

When Diane's egg pick-up time is decided, Michael is informed, for he will be required to provide a semen sample a few hours later.

Egg pick-up

For the pick-up to succeed, three things are required—accurate timing so that eggs are sufficiently mature, accessibility of the ovaries to the laparoscope, and a good egg collection technique.

Women having an egg pick-up by the technique of laparoscopy are given a general anaesthetic, for although it is possible to perform laparoscopy under local anaesthesia, the egg pick-up procedure is more complex and the possible application of local anaesthesia is still being explored. As pregnancies have occurred following relatively prolonged general anaesthesia, it is not thought that the anaesthetic affects the eggs.

Normally when a laparoscopy is performed solely to examine the ovaries, two incisions are made in the abdomen. A cut, a few millimeters long is made in the umbilicus (navel), and a telescope-like instrument with its own light attached—the laparoscope—is introduced so that the ovaries can be viewed.

The second puncture site is usually made in the lower abdomen along the hair line and a fine forceps is passed through. This allows the pelvic organs to be manipulated and positioned appropriately.

When a laparoscopy for the purpose of picking up eggs is being carried out, a third puncture may be made between the first and second incisions (see Figure 8). This enables the surgeon to pass a Teflon®-coated needle into each mature follicle and remove the fluid and the egg it contains. Alternatively, a right-angled off-set laparoscope is used, requiring only two puncture sites.

By looking through the laparoscope held in one hand, and manipulating each ovary into various positions with the other, the surgeon can identify any ripe follicles. These look like button mushrooms and are 1.5 to 2.5 cm in size. They usually have a thin wall, through which the fluid inside is visible.

Each follicle is a delicate structure, so gentleness is essential at this stage of the procedure. The needle is passed through the wall of the follicle as slowly and as carefully as possible in order to prevent fluid leakage or damage to the egg.

By means of a vacuum pressure device that the surgeon operates

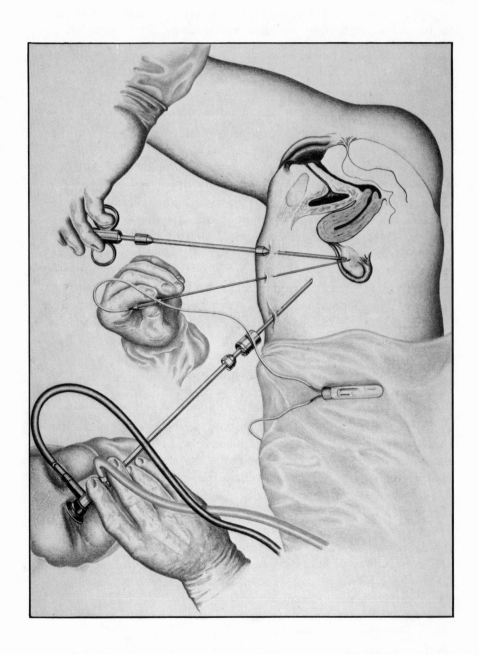

Figure 8 (opposite). The technique of egg pick-up: a laparoscope is placed through the umbilicus to view the ovary. A second instrument is passed through the abdomen lower down, to hold the ovary. A needle is inserted between these to suck the fluid containing the egg from the ovary.

by foot, the fluid is sucked from the follicle through the needle and placed in a flat glass dish. The amount of fluid is usually about five to fifteen milliliters and is the color of straw. The egg itself within the fluid is only one-tenth of a millimeter in size and is invisible to the naked eye. However, as it is usually surrounded by mucus and a layer of cells about one millimeter in diameter, the whole complex may be seen as a tiny white speck in the fluid.

As rapidly as possible, this fluid is taken to a laboratory near the operating room, and a scientist or a specially trained laboratory technician immediately examines it under high magnification.

As soon as the egg is identified, a message is sent through the intercom to the surgeon in the operating room. The surgeon stops examining that follicle for the egg and proceeds to look for other mature follicles.

Sometimes the egg is not collected because it is attached to the wall of the follicle and is not in the free fluid that has been removed. When the technician reports that no egg is present in the fluid collected, the surgeon injects fluid into the follicle until it reaches its original size. The fluid is then sucked out in the hope that any egg that has adhered to the wall of the follicle will become detached.

Eggs collected by this technique of flushing the follicle are less likely to be fully mature, because one of the natural changes that occurs prior to ovulation is that the egg becomes free-floating in the fluid of the follicle. Nevertheless, pregnancies have followed follicle

Figure 9. Aspiration needle used to collect the fluid containing the egg from the ovary. The needle is coated with Teflon® to prevent the egg from sticking.

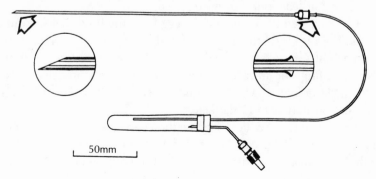

50mm

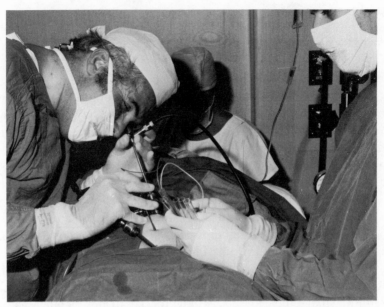

Figure 10. Laparoscopy with glass tubes ready for collecting ovarian fluid that contains the egg(s).

flushing. If an egg cannot be found after several flushings, the search is abandoned.

Sometimes when the laparoscopy is performed, ovulation has already occurred. This is recognized by the fact that the follicle or follicles previously identified—using ultrasound—have burst.

In this situation, all is not lost. The egg may drop from the ovary into the pouch behind the uterus, whence it can sometimes be collected. Two things are done. The ruptured follicle is flushed, as the egg may still be stuck within it, and the fluid from the pouch behind the uterus is sucked out and examined.

Advances in the technique of egg collection and the increasing skill of the surgeons have resulted in a situation where, in nine out of ten patients, at least one egg is collected.

The next step is to separate the egg from the fluid that surrounds it. If the fluid is clear, this is not difficult. But if blood is present, and particularly if a clot has formed around the egg and its surrounding cells, separating one from the other is not easy. Fortunately, the egg has some elasticity and will withstand minor distortion. But any strong manipulation may lead to damage.

It is possible to collect eggs without an operation and general anaesthetic. A needle can be guided to the ovary using ultrasound pictures and local anaesthesia. This technique, which is still under

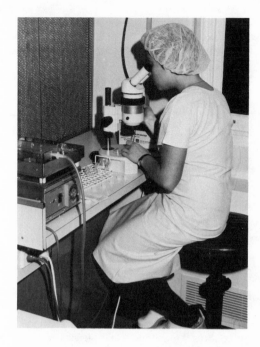

Figure 11. Scientist checks that an egg has been collected during the laparoscopy. An ordinary microscope is used.

development, would simplify treatment. A pregnancy in Sweden has followed the needle-ultrasonic technique of egg collection.

Egg culture

Once the egg is free, it is placed as quickly as possible in the culture fluid, which in turn is placed in an incubator. This provides suitable conditions for sustaining the health of the egg; temperature and humidity are controlled precisely and a clean environment is assured over the surface of the culture fluid.

For the next five to twelve hours, the egg is left undisturbed in the hope that it will attain a state of maturity similar to that which occurs at the time of ovulation.

If many eggs are collected, a woman taking part in the Queen Victoria Medical Centre program may consider donating one or more eggs to another woman who cannot produce eggs. Then IVF is carried out using sperm cells from the recipient's partner. In the U.S., donation of eggs has not yet occurred.

Michael has been advised not to ejaculate for several days before the probable day of the egg pick-up in order to produce a good supply

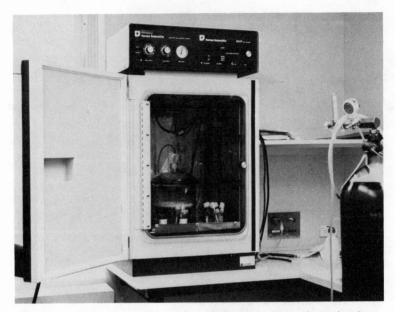

Figure 12. Incubator in which eggs mature and early embryo development takes place. The incubator controls the chemical and physical environment surrounding the fluid in which the eggs are cultured.

of sperm cells. Two hours after Diane's successful operation, he collects a semen sample by masturbation in a room close to the laboratory.

Male partners often have difficulty collecting a sample in such unusual and stressful circumstances (see Chapter 6), and in such cases their mates are asked to assist. This may be difficult because of the woman's recent anaesthesia, but it has the benefit of involving both partners in a critical step of the conception.

It would be preferable if the semen could be collected after sexual intercourse, as this would incorporate the act of bodily love in the procedure. However, there are two difficulties to be overcome in this respect. Collection of the semen in a condom may lead to deterioration of the sperm cells, so a special type of condom is necessary. Secondly, some women feel sick, drowsy, or otherwise uncomfortable a few hours after the laparoscopy and so would find it difficult to have intercourse at this time. Teams working in this field are attempting to develop alternative methods of collecting semen.

In order for sperm cells to be capable of penetrating the egg, they have to undergo a change from the state they are in at the time of ejaculation. This change, called *capacitation*, normally occurs as the sperm cells pass through the female genital tract and involves the shedding of the outer coat of the sperm head.

68

Capacitation has a number of other benefits. It results in increased sperm cell activity, and they therefore move more vigorously. Also, the chemicals released during capacitation may assist in sperm cell penetration of the layer of cells and the coat surrounding the egg.

In the human, inducing capacitation is quite simple, in contrast to the situation in many other species. It is achieved by washing the sperm cells twice in a simple solution and leaving them in culture fluid for one to two hours. Then the sperm cells are examined under a microscope to ensure that they are still active, and those required for fertilization are collected. This involves a relatively simple selection procedure, as the most healthy and active sperm cells tend to be concentrated in the upper part of the culture fluid.

Fertilization

About 50,000 sperm cells are placed with the egg, in the procedure known as *insemination*.

The egg and the sperm cells are then returned to the incubator with the expectation that a single sperm cell will penetrate the egg. This is the first of a series of steps in the process of fertilization.

The sperm cell passes through the outer layer of cells and mucus surrounding the egg, and then through the coat and substance of the

Figure 13. Sperm consist of three parts: a large head containing genetic material, a long tail for propulsion, and a small middle section that, like a battery, provides energy for movement.

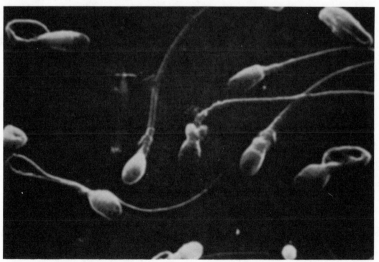

egg. This normally takes several hours and requires the action of chemical substances from the sperm cell together with its own physical thrust from movement of the tail.

As soon as one sperm cell has passed into the core of the egg, a barrier to further sperm cell entry is usually created by chemicals released by the egg. If more than one sperm cell enters, fertilization may be abnormal or unsuccessful, or embryo development may proceed abnormally.

This is one theoretical disadvantage of the *in vitro* fertilization procedure—since a larger number of sperm cells are in a position to enter the egg than in the orthodox situation—as it would seem more likely that several sperm cells could enter simultaneously, before the barrier to further sperm cell entry became effective. This occurrence would lead to abnormalities.

However, since the number of sperm cells placed with the egg has been reduced from 500,000 to 50,000, this has not been a problem.

The result of penetration by the sperm cell is that its genetic material combines with the genetic material of the egg, thus providing the blueprint that is essential for the development of a new human life.

Embryo growth and assessment

As described in Chapter 1, the embryo so formed moves through a series of cell divisions, and about forty-eight hours after insemination, it has grown from one cell to eight.

The quality or health of the embryo is judged by the speed at which it develops, as well as by its appearance. In a normal embryo, the cells are regular in outline and approximately equal in size. Irregularity of cells or distortion of shape indicates abnormality. Experience shows that an embryo with an abnormal appearance or very slow growth no longer has the potential to form a human life. Since it no longer has this potential, it is certified as dead and, as in the case of adult material in which death has occurred with no apparent cause, an examination may be carried out to try to determine the reason.

The information gained is not always conclusive, but sometimes it is possible to determine the cause of abnormal embryo growth.

Early in the history of the Melbourne program, embryo transfers were carried out at the eight- or sixteen-cell stage of development. It is now clear that the uterus will accept embryos consisting of one, two, or four cells, and pregnancies have followed at these early stages.

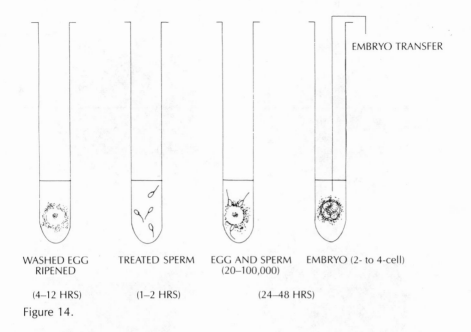

WASHED EGG   TREATED SPERM   EGG AND SPERM   EMBRYO (2- to 4-cell)
RIPENED   (20–100,000)

(4–12 HRS)   (1–2 HRS)   (24–48 HRS)

Figure 14.

This early transfer has some advantages. It avoids a prolonged period in the culture fluid, components of which may deteriorate with time, and once the transfer is made, the possibility of environmental contamination of the embryo culture fluid or the occurrence of an accident affecting the embryo is removed.

It is still uncertain whether the human embryo should ideally be transferred at the one-, two-, four-, eight-, or sixteen-cell stage, and only careful studies will determine this.

If fertilization does not occur, the egg is studied to find out why and, whenever possible, an explanation is offered to the couple concerned. Sometimes a cause is evident, and steps to overcome the problem may be taken during the next treatment attempt.

The best chance of becoming pregnant is achieved if four or more mature eggs are removed from the ovaries and several embryos develop.

In the case of Diane and Michael, three eggs are picked up, but only one embryo develops. During fertilization and growth of their embryo, they are kept informed of progress.

The policy of fertilizing all mature eggs sometimes results in the formation of four or more embryos. In this situation, both the couple and the treatment team face an ethical quandary.

The couple may wish to have two, three or four embryos transferred, but not for example, five, because of the very small chance of quintuplets' developing. In general, couples are advised to accept three embryos

71

Figure 15.

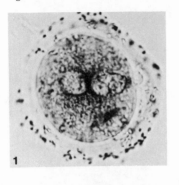

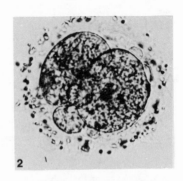

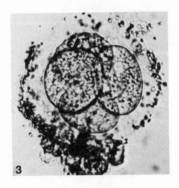

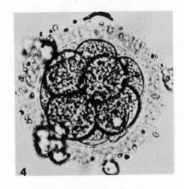

(1): single-cell embryo. Two small round bodies are seen within the embryo. One contains genetic material of the sperm and the other genetic material of the egg. The sperm can no longer be seen within the egg. Eighteen hours have elapsed since this sperm was united with the egg.

(3): four-cell embryo (forty-two hours old). The four cells are still contained within the coat of the egg.

(2): two-cell embryo (thirty hours old)—the two cells are of equal size and rounded. The small round body—the polar body—contains discarded genetic material.

(4): eight-cell embryo (fifty-six hours old)—stage of development normally attained while egg is still in the Fallopian tube. Embryos are transferred anywhere between the one- to eight-cell stage. In our experience, transfers are most successful at the two- to four-cell stage.

as, even with this number, the chance of twins is small and of triplets, remote. In the United States, all fertilized, cleaving embryos are re-implanted.

Although twins are associated with slightly increased risks, such as premature labor and a higher mortality rate, the prospect of two

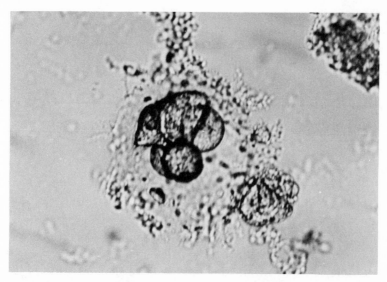

Figure 16. Frozen four-cell embryo appears distorted because it loses water and shrinks during freezing. A chemical preservative is used to prevent damage to the embryo.

babies rather than one is attractive to most couples. Having been infertile for some years, they appreciate that this may be their only chance of establishing a family.

The dilemma remains about what to do with the extra embryos.

At the Queen Victoria Medical Centre, embryos are frozen in liquid nitrogen for use by the couple at a later date. The reasons for adopting this procedure are discussed in Chapter 8. In the United States, embryo freezing (cryopreservation) is not generally accepted or practiced.

Although freezing and thawing embryos has not been followed by completed pregnancies at the time of writing, there is reason for cautious optimism as several eight-cell embryos have grown until a later stage of development after this procedure.

With animals, the freezing and thawing of embryos has been achieved on thousands of occasions, leading to the birth of perfectly healthy sheep, mice, and calves.

The embryo transfer

Although the transfer of the embryo to the uterus is a very critical procedure, the technique is reasonably simple.

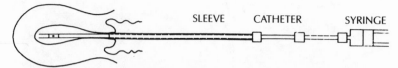

SLEEVE   CATHETER   SYRINGE

Figure 17. Transfer of embryo to uterus: inside a small drop of fluid, the embryo is injected from the catheter into the uterus.

One to two days after the sperm cells are placed with the egg, a scientist decides whether the embryo is normal in appearance and growing well enough for a transfer to take place.

The embryo is growing normally, and an hour before the proposed time of the transfer Diane is offered a tranquilizer. Although it is a pity to dampen feelings at this time, some patients are overanxious and find it difficult to relax sufficiently to enable the doctor to achieve a smooth, gentle transfer. It is also possible that anxiety may make the uterus more active by stimulating the release of certain hormones, and this may increase the risk of embryo expulsion.

At one time, patients were given a drug to block uterine activity in the hope that this would improve the success of embryo transfer, but this was not effective so the practice has been abandoned.

The embryo transfer takes place in the operating room, in a bid

Figure 18. The embryo transfer: the potential mother lies on her back, and the doctor and scientist place the embryo back into the uterus as gently as possible. The male partner and the nurse talk to the patient during this painless procedure.

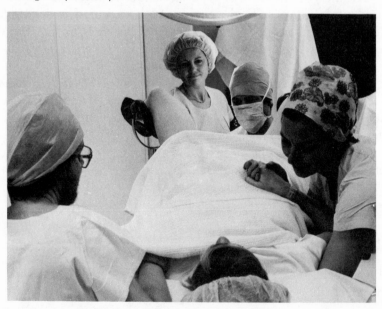

74

to reduce the risk of infection during the procedure. This location has the obvious disadvantage of being more clinical than that occurring at the time of embryo implantation under orthodox conditions.

In order to partially offset this disadvantage, Michael is encouraged to be present. Both he and Diane feel that this is the most human point in their attempt to have a child. They are together, fully aware of what is happening, and for them this moment compensates in some degree for the absence of the sexual act.

In a room close to the operating room, the embryo is placed in a tiny drop of fluid that is transferred to a fine tube about one millimeter in diameter. Although placement of the embryo in this drop of fluid requires considerable skill, it is extremely rare that an embryo is damaged during the procedure: The scientists practice the technique on mouse embryos until they are expert enough to handle human embryos.

It is important that subsequent events occur as quickly and as gently as possible. An embryo in such a tiny drop of fluid may be affected adversely by cold air or evaporation of the fluid that surrounds it, and this could lead to critical changes in its chemistry.

While the embryo is made ready, Diane lies on her back with her legs in stirrups and covered by drapes. The doctor inserts a speculum—the metal instrument shaped to fit the vagina—and exposes the cervix. The position and size of the uterus are checked in order to determine the best method for passing the tube containing the embryo into it. Any excess fluid on the cervix is removed because, if this is introduced into the cervix as the catheter is passed, it may stick to the embryo and prevent it from implanting in the uterus.

The scientist is alerted that all is ready, and the embryo is brought into the operating room. Working together, the doctor and scientist pass the tube or catheter through the vagina and then through the cervix a short distance into the uterus.

The best place for the release of the embryo is not known for certain, but it seems reasonable that this should occur at about the place where the Fallopian tube meets the uterus, which is a half to one centimeter from the top of the uterus.

This position is accurately determined from a measurement of the length of the uterus made during an ultrasound scan earlier in the cycle or during a preliminary laparoscopy or endometrial biopsy. By marking the distance on the catheter and subtracting a centimeter, the surgeon is assured of reasonably correct placement.

The catheter is passed slowly and gently, as any forceful manipulation against the wall of the uterus could cause bleeding or stimulate uterine activity. Either could thwart the transfer attempt.

If the catheter sticks as it passes through the cervix, it is manipulated in various directions in an attempt to find a clear passage.

The technique of embryo transfer requires practice, experience, and patience, as the natural tendency is to want to complete the procedure as quickly as possible in order to protect the embryo.

Often, the catheter is passed inside a guiding sheath that helps to direct it through the cervix and uterus. In recent years, also, improvements to catheters (see Chapter 3) have resulted in easier transfers. A surgeon may choose from a range of catheters, since one may be more suitable than others in a particular situation.

Women who have had a vaginal delivery previously have an advantage here, for childbirth dilates the cervix to some extent, and the catheter thus passes more easily into the uterus.

A trial transfer is sometimes carried out before the treatment cycle. This has several advantages: The patient becomes acquainted with the procedure and is often more confident and less anxious about it, and if difficulties arise during the trial transfer, the cause of the problem may be identified and preventive measures may be possible at the time of the actual transfer. For example, very anxious patients in whom the vagina contracts during examination can be given an epidural anaesthetic. Or if the catheter will not pass easily through the cervix, the patient can have a dilatation of the cervix before the treatment cycle. This involves a day in the hospital and a general anaesthetic during the month before the treatment cycle and results in an easier transfer.

In Diane's case, the embryo transfer proves to be quite difficult, and the embryo is returned to the laboratory and placed in culture fluid before another transfer is attempted with a different catheter. Pregnancies have occurred after such a sequence of events.

Sometimes the transfer is impossible or doomed to failure. For example, if bleeding occurs in the uterus, it may form a clot around the embryo, preventing implantation; or else the embryo may be washed through the cervix with the blood.

It may be impossible to pass the catheter through the cervix. In this circumstance, there are several alternatives: Either the embryo is replaced in the culture fluid and another attempt is made the next day using anaesthesia and dilating the cervix, or it is frozen for transfer at a later date. The only other options are for the couple to donate it to another couple or to attempt transfer through the top of the uterus by means of laparoscopy and insertion of a needle into the uterine cavity.

In Diane's case, the second attempt is successful, and as soon as

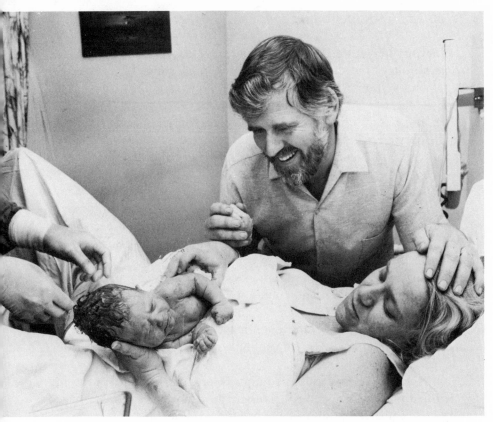

Figure 19. Birth of Pippin Brennan (father Len, mother Jan) at the Queen Victoria Medical Centre, July 1981. This was one of many births during 1981—indicating that the techniques had become more reliable.

the catheter tip is in the desired position within the uterus, the embryo is released.

The catheter is withdrawn slowly in order to minimize the chance of the embryo's moving along an artificial track left by it (e.g., a slight depression in the tissue where the catheter has pressed).

A disadvantage of transferring the embryo through the cervix is that the catheter disrupts the plug of mucus that would tend normally to assist in the retention of the embryo.

After the transfer procedure, the catheter is inspected in the laboratory under the microscope to ensure that the embryo has indeed been delivered into the patient.

Care and assessment after transfer

Following the transfer, Diane is lifted gently from the operating table onto a trolley, and she is then taken back to the ward.

The best approach to patient care following embryo transfer is uncertain.

In the conventional situation, of course, no special care is taken, and embryos are thought to implant after three days in the uterus. But because the mucus plug of the cervix is punctured, Diane is advised to rest on her side for four hours before going home, and she is discouraged from long-distance travel during the next few days.

Couples are advised not to have sexual intercourse until tests indicate whether pregnancy has occurred. These tests—on the seventh, tenth, twelfth, and fourteenth days after the transfer—also indicate whether the pregnancy is likely to continue.

Low levels of pregnancy hormones are associated with an increased risk of natural abortion, and couples are warned of this possibility.

Both in the natural system of conception and the test-tube procedure, abortions occur most often before or around the time of the next period. Women in the conventional situation are usually unaware of such abortions.

Once the pregnancy has continued for eight weeks following *in vitro* fertilization and embryo transfer, the chances of a miscarriage are very similar to those in the conventional situation.

In cases where eggs are not fertilized, an embryo does not grow, or a pregnancy does not occur after the transfer procedure, it is important for couples to see their doctor so that the situation can be discussed and a decision made about a further treatment attempt.

In the Monash/QVMC/Epworth program, couples usually have three or four treatment attempts, although some have continued and become pregnant after five or six treatments.

The time interval between treatments is best decided by couples after discussion with their doctor. Some couples prefer to have the attempts within a short period of time so that the matter can be dealt with as quickly as possible. They can then organize their lives according to whether a pregnancy has or has not occurred. Others prefer to space the attempts at yearly intervals either to recuperate from each attempt, to save money for the next attempt, or to improve their chances of success—assuming that the success rate of the procedure will improve each year.

Deciding when to abandon treatment—such as if the couple is being adversely affected emotionally or if eggs are difficult to collect

Figure 20.

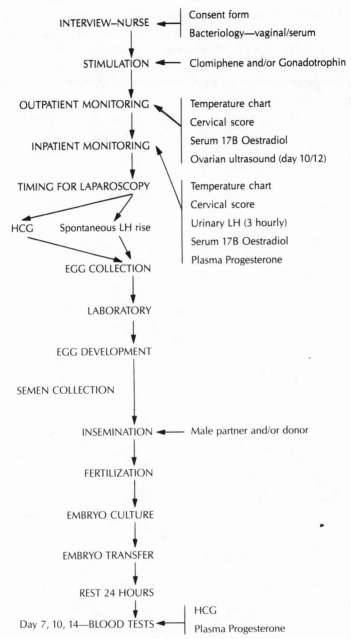

or don't fertilize—is a difficult decision, especially after a lengthy period of treatment in which high hopes are invested. In making the decision, partners should be clear about the treatments that have been attempted and whether any other treatment has a reasonable chance of success.

During the treatment, partners may become overwrought, and sometimes it is a good idea to postpone the treatment until emotional and physical energy is restored.

When all possible treatments have been offered, it is important that couples understand that this is so, and to face the reality of not being able to have their own children.

6

Practical Problems

Couples taking part in the test-tube-baby program may face significant social, financial, emotional, and physical difficulties.

The waiting list

The present waiting period for the program in Melbourne is two years, and more than 2000 couples are on the waiting list at the Epworth/ Queen Victoria Medical Centre alone. There are also lengthy waiting periods for other programs in Australia and in other countries.

Some couples who join the program never reach the treatment stage. Some with unknown causes of infertility may become pregnant while on the waiting list, and others change their minds about pursuing the treatment, perhaps because of a change in social circumstance, marital problems, or increasing age.

The long waiting period is unavoidable, and couples who feel desperate about their infertility may find the delay agonizing. The stress that this imposes, as well as ways to resolve it, is discussed later in this chapter.

In the meantime, possible alternative treatments such as further tubal flushing, a repeat attempt at tubal repair, or the use of fertility drugs are likely to be considered.

The lengthy waiting period and the uncertainty of success means that the possibility of adoption should be considered as early as possible.

Rarely is an adopted baby available without a wait of two or three years, and sometimes it may be more like five or six years; some couples become too old to qualify and thus are never able to become adoptive parents.

Now that the success rate of the test-tube-baby program is reliably established and the procedure is recognized as a valuable treatment for many infertile couples, it is hoped that waiting lists will become matters of historical interest. Once rebates for the treatment are more comprehensive—covering a greater number of procedures, such as initial use of hormones, hormone measurements, egg pick-up, sperm preparation, and embryo transfer—it should be possible to expand programs to meet the demand. (No rebates at all are available in the United States.)

Selection priority is another aspect of the waiting list that may cause concern.

It has been suggested that couples who are willing to pay more should be given preference, particularly as most IVF teams are short of money. Our current policy is to accept all patients who have passed the selection procedure according to medical indications, providing they are married and under the age of forty. Factors taken into account during selection are outlined in Chapter 4, and once patients have been assessed they are placed on the waiting list in order of application.

Occasionally a special group of patients is given priority in order to settle a matter of uncertainty that may benefit significant numbers of infertile patients. Currently, for example, twelve men with low sperm counts are being studied to determine whether there is a place for the procedure to treat this problem. Such research groups are kept as small as possible to test the theory under scrutiny while minimizing disturbance to the general flow of the program.

Patients are placed on the waiting list in order of completion of an entry form, and it is worth checking, a few months after joining the program, that your name has been added to the list. At this time, couples can also request an updated estimate of how long it will be before treatment is likely to begin. Some programs give priority to couples who have no children.

Absence from work or family

A woman may have a problem if work or family commitments make it difficult to obtain leave of absence when her turn for treatment arrives. It may be possible to negotiate several months during the year when leave from work can be granted. This could depend on the availability of others to carry on the job, or the general workload that it involves. These months can then be discussed with the treatment team to see if an arrangement can be made to suit all concerned.

Sometimes a leave of absence does not fit in with menstrual cycles, and other unpredictable events may occur, but by trial and error it is usually possible to find an opportunity for treatment.

A further complication is that most teams go into recess for a time each year. Our own vacation break is only for one week. Unless the team is very large, breaks are unavoidable, and they may be important in providing an opportunity for planning improvements to the program for the following year.

During the treatment cycle it is necessary to be available for blood tests from at least Day 8 onward, and the hospital stay is from five to seven days. Many women stop work for about three weeks during the treatment cycle, although others prefer to remain as busy as possible.

Financial aspects

The cost of the procedure depends on whether the service is carried out in a public or private clinic.

In the Monash/QVMC/Epworth program, egg pick-ups and embryo transfers are performed at a private hospital, as it has not been possible to organize the procedure in the public hospital system. A similar situation exists in the clinic of Drs. Edwards and Steptoe in England, and the Drs. Jones' clinic in the United States.

In Melbourne, this arrangement means that patients need to save the total cost of the procedure—which amounts to $3000 to $3500 for each treatment attempt. In the United States, the cost of treatment varies between approximately $3500 and $8000. In Melbourne, patients have the option of joining a health-insurance organization and receiving a substantial reimbursement. No such plan is available in the United States.

Couples who join the Monash/QVMC/Epworth program also face a surcharge for both the laparoscopy and the embryo transfer if they get to these stages of the treatment. These surcharges amount to nearly $600 and they help keep the programs operating.

Although medical costs account for the major part of the financial outlay, there are other expenses worth bearing in mind.

In assessing whether they can afford the *in vitro* fertilization and embryo transfer treatment, couples need to consider the hidden costs of travel, accommodation, and pharmacy bills (for instance, for fertility drugs), as well as any loss of personal income of either partner. Added loss of income occurs when the husband travels with his wife to give support. Programs in the United States are for the most part restricted to large cities or special centers.

Although the cost of each treatment attempt may seem relatively high, it is comparable to the cost of a tubal repair and is considerably less than the cost of rearing a child should a pregnancy occur.

Stress

The test-tube-baby procedure is a treatment with extraordinary benefits balanced against high personal costs.

Any type of infertility investigation and treatment imposes many stresses on an already stressful situation. Some forms of stress are common to all types of infertility treatment; others are peculiar to *in vitro* fertilization and embryo transfer.

Some of the causes of these stresses include: a state of suspense during long periods of waiting, waiting on lists, waiting for results at the various stages of treatment, waiting after a failed attempt, waiting and perhaps grieving for some months before the next attempt; inconvenience, embarrassment, pain, and discussion about subjects that are usually intimate and private; anxiety about doing the right thing in a climate of public debate about the procedure; concern that time is passing with the loss of possibly fertile years; reliance on the expertise and consideration of the team members.

In the test-tube procedure in particular, the usual one-to-one relationship between the doctor and patient is altered, and several doctors may be involved in care-taking at different stages of the treatment. This is because teams are organized on a roster basis in order to cover the twenty-four-hours-a-day, seven-days-a-week treatment schedule. Furthermore, within the program there is specialization, for some doctors are very skillful at performing egg pick-ups, so this procedure is concentrated in their hands; others are better at determining the complicated hormone stimulation and fertility drug schedules and keep a careful watch on these.

This "team treatment" can have disadvantages, as a doctor who is expert in one area of treatment may not fully understand other aspects in a particular situation. Should couples feel that something has been overlooked, it is important that they question the team members in order to clarify the situation.

If couples can understand the limitations of team members, and of existing knowledge, they will be in a better position to cope with disappointments and failures if the treatment does not work.

Emotional tensions peak at times of egg pick-up and embryo transfer. Peaks of hope and excitement may be followed by troughs of depression, an exhausting way to live. This may be followed by the emotionally draining process of adjusting to alternatives.

Problems in the couple's relationship. The original motivation for a pregnancy may be complicated by issues such as guilt about being the infertile partner, resentment that the other partner is not fertile, or dismay at a partner's preoccupation with having a child.

Having to make numerous decisions about commencing and continuing investigations and treatments, and about when to stop. There may be decisions during the treatment itself that the couple will need to face squarely. For example, in the situation where a problem involving sperm cells may be contributing to infertility, the couple may be asked whether they want the eggs to be fertilized with the male partner's sperm cells only, those from a donor, or both. And if embryos develop from both the partner's and the donor's sperm cells, should one or both embryos be transferred?

Or if a donor egg becomes available at the same time as an unsuccessful egg pick-up, would the couple wish to have it added to the male's sperm cells in a bid to achieve embryo formation and a subsequent pregnancy?

Another decision may be necessary if as many as five or six embryos develop. How many embryos would the couple wish to have transferred?

And if a pregnancy does occur, what of publicity? Public relations officers of hospitals associated with the test-tube-baby programs will present one viewpoint, but the final decision should be one with which both partners are happy.

Worry about the social and psychological implications for a child conceived through in vitro fertilization. Parents may worry that their child's unconventional beginning may have adverse effects. However, if parents' attitudes toward the nature of the conception are positive and open, it seems unlikely that children will suffer psychological damage. There is always the possibility that other children and adults with whom the child comes into contact may make unfavorable comments to them. Certainly at various stages of growing up, one is very sensitive to such remarks, and parents should be prepared to protect and reassure their child if such events occur.

Parents may worry about informing their child of the role of the test-tube procedure in his or her conception, and because of the publicity surrounding the early births, it would seem almost impossible that parents would not need to discuss the part played by the test-tube-baby procedure. But as pregnancies in IVF programs increase in number, such publicity is likely to diminish, and parents will have more choice in this matter.

Social workers have described crises in the lives of adopted children who, on realizing that their adoptive parents are not their biological parents, desperately wish to establish their parentage. This type of crisis is unlikely to occur unless donor sperm cells or a donor egg is used during the *in vitro* fertilization procedure.

Indeed, far from a life crisis, it is possible that children born with the help of the procedure will have very positive feelings of self-esteem and self-importance, given the special steps that their parents took to ensure their existence.

Some people become sick or emotionally and physically drained as a result of stress. Others feel somewhat stimulated and regard difficulties as a challenge. The stress response, innate in many species, is an emergency survival reaction that prepares the body for "flight or fight," but in the situation of infertility treatment, most of the stresses faced cannot be dealt with in this way. The body is prepared for action but is often unable to act. It thus remains in a temporary "alarm" state that may eventually result in exhaustion.

In some cases, it may be better to defer treatment for a time or perhaps take a vacation.

Aware of these stresses, many test-tube-baby teams now include skilled counselors with whom couples can talk through their problems and the stress they face and discuss various methods of coming to terms with the situation.

Self-help groups for infertile couples and those taking part in IVF programs also provide valuable support.

Masturbation

Masturbation to obtain a semen sample poses problems for some men taking part in the program.

The physical difficulties of masturbating to produce a sample have been largely overlooked, perhaps because studies of sexual behavior have found repeatedly that most men masturbate. However, they do so at a time and place that suits their mood, not in a hospital room to produce a sample on the crucial day that eggs have been collected from their partners. It is hardly surprising that the latter situation often triggers considerable anxiety and interferes with sexual performance—causing impotence or incomplete or ineffective ejaculation.

It would be helpful if the environment of the hospital room where the sample is collected were more relaxed, but this is not always feasible. The presence of the partner can be valuable, but this may prove to be impossible as she may be recovering after the egg pick-up procedure.

Difficulties with masturbation can often be overcome by practice. In one training program based on behavioral therapy techniques, the man practices masturbating while imagining that he is in the situation on the day of the egg pick-up. He draws a mental picture of his partner in the operating room and—with several eggs collected—it is now up to him to produce a semen sample in a small room close to the operating room. These images tend to produce considerable anxiety concerning masturbation, but if masturbation can be performed repeatedly with this picture in mind, he learns to overcome the anxiety. When the day comes, he usually finds the actual situation much easier to cope with.

Another way to improve masturbation performance is to heighten the erotic state in an attempt to overcome anxiety. This can be achieved by imagining sexual fantasies that appeal to the particular male, or by viewing pictures of exciting and beautiful women.

Men who cannot learn to masturbate easily or with consistent success or who are particularly anxious about masturbating on the day of the egg pick-up can provide a semen sample prior to this day and the sample is frozen and stored. The fact that a back-up sample is available tends to reduce anxiety and improve the production of the preferred fresh sample on the day of the egg pick-up. (Fertilization is more likely with fresh than thawed sperm cells.)

The words of one woman in the program express eloquently the effect of an inability to masturbate on the appointed day: "There's nothing in the world like waking up from an *in vitro* operation and finding that you have a normal healthy egg and a normal healthy husband, but no sperm. I felt dreadfully disappointed and angry at the situation, and also very ashamed of myself that I had put my husband through such a humiliating experience."

Legal protection for the child and parents

At present, the law does not provide adequate protection for, and fails to define satisfactorily, the relationship between the principal participants in the test-tube-baby program—that is, the clinicians, the prospective parents, and the future child. On August 10, 1981, an editorial in the Melbourne daily newspaper *The Age* put it thus:

> Like the hare and the tortoise, science and the law run a permanently unequal race. While science moves in dazzling leaps and pirouettes, weaving wonder and miracles, the law plods sedately behind and collects the dust. It is sometimes a very long plod.

A number of aspects of the test-tube-baby program urgently require legal clarification.

1. The area of compensation for pre-conception and pre-birth injuries. The legal rights regarding compensation for a child born disabled as a result of the procedure are not clear. And if compensation is to be made available, who should bear the burden of payment? If placed upon teams, would medical initiatives in this area cease? Currently, a child born disabled in Australia as a result of something done, or omitted, during the procedure would be entitled only to compensation if it could be established that the act or omission by the scientist, technician, or some other person constituted actionable negligence. This is not an easy matter to prove. Whereas in a procedure that is well tried and established it is relatively easy to prove that a departure from the regular method that resulted in injury or damage constitutes actionable negligence, the test-tube procedure is still in a state of development and change.

2. The right of a child to bring an action against a clinician who fails to detect fetal abnormality.

3. That embryo transfer does not constitute a type of abortion, even if the operation is not successful and the embryo dies in the process.

4. The rights of partners whose embryo has been frozen and who now disagree about the future of their embryo. Both might seek custody or one might wish it to be discarded. In whose favor should this difficult issue be resolved, given the essentially equal nature of their contributions?

5. The future of a frozen embryo should both prospective parents die—for example, in an accident. Should the embryo become the property of the next of kin, or go into a pool to be used for the benefit of other infertile couples?

7
The Pregnancy

The number of babies born with the help of *in vitro* fertilization and embryo transfer is still relatively small—about 300, more than one hundred of whom have been born in Melbourne. Thus the information available about pregnancies is limited. Undoubtedly much useful information will emerge during the next few years as the number of babies conceived in the laboratory increases.

To date no major problems have arisen, but several aspects of the pregnancies are of interest.

Obstetrical complications

Obstetrical complications may be slightly more common than usual because of the age of patients when they become pregnant. Most are in their thirties or forties.

Sex of the baby

In Melbourne, initially more girls than boys were delivered, but the trend has changed and no difference in sex ratio of births is now apparent.

Fetal malformation

A major area of concern is whether the incidence of fetal malformation is higher than, the same as, or lower than the 3 percent rate of malformations occurring in naturally reproducing couples.

It has been suggested that Down's syndrome (Mongolism) will occur more often. This disorder, due to a chromosomal abnormality,

89

can be detected in about the fourteenth week of pregnancy. As the usual genetic changes that produce this syndrome occur in the egg before it is collected by laparoscopy, it seems unlikely that the test-tube-baby procedure would markedly increase this hazard.

The other type of abnormality that is theoretically more likely is the penetration of the egg by more than one sperm cell, causing a situation known as *polyspermy*. In the few known births that have occurred in this century following polyspermy, abnormalities are severe. It is likely that continuing pregnancies do not occur often because polyspermy tends to be followed by failure of fertilization, abnormal fertilization, or an abnormal embryo that is aborted naturally within the first few days or weeks of the pregnancy. Thus, even if there is a small risk of this situation's occurring, it is unlikely to be a practical problem.

Of the first 120 babies born in Australia up to November 1983 only one had a defect, and this was a heart abnormality that was corrected surgically. It seems unlikely that this defect was due to the test-tube procedure, but any statement about the likelihood of fetal malformation will be conclusive only when hundreds or thousands of test-tube babies have been delivered. However, at this time the rate of major malformations following the test-tube procedure is lower than that occuring in the natural system.

Because of concern about the possibility of fetal malformation, the growth and hormone output of the fetus is monitored carefully during the pregnancy. The measurements following laboratory conceptions are identical to those following orthodox conceptions. As a result of this finding, it is unlikely that specific tests related to fetal growth or production of hormones will be necessary in the future.

Most patients wish to have at least one ultrasound scan to confirm that they are pregnant and to be reassured that the fetus appears to be normal.

In addition, one other test is offered to pregnant patients. This is amniocentesis, which involves the sampling and testing of the amniotic fluid that bathes the fetus. This enables detection of central nervous system defects, such as spina bifida, or chromosomal abnormalities, such as Down's syndrome.

Couples need to recognize that there is a slight risk of miscarriage (about one in 200) associated with amniocentesis. Another important matter for consideration is whether couples would act on the information from the test. If they would not, then it is pointless to subject the pregnancy to the risk of a miscarriage. More than half of our couples decide not to have an amniocentesis because they are unwilling to have a therapeutic abortion, even if an abnormality is detected.

The amniocentesis is carried out at twelve to fourteen weeks of pregnancy, and the results may take several weeks to process, so therapeutic abortion can be offered only when the woman is more than four months pregnant. Abortion at this stage presents a risk to the mother particularly in relation to infection, hemorrhage, or damage to the cervix, and this should be taken into account when deciding about having an amniocentesis.

None of our patients, up to the end of 1983, have had a therapeutic abortion following the test-tube procedure.

Psychological problems

Psychological problems during the pregnancy may be more common than usual as, naturally enough, couples are more than usually anxious about their baby.

These problems often cannot be resolved until the birth, but regular visits to the doctor to check that all is well can prove invaluable.

Choice of doctor and hospital

During the first few years of the program in Melbourne, we are asking couples to accept delivery by specialists who understand the *in vitro* fertilization and embryo transfer procedures. This enables detailed records to be collected that are essential for research purposes, such as follow-up studies. It is intended that all children resulting from the procedure in Australia will be followed up on for some years in order to ascertain their emotional, physical, and intellectual development.

Now that more than one hundred babies have been delivered, the choice of the obstetrician and hospital has been liberalized. It is likely, however, that because of the couples' increased age and history of infertility, specialist care will always be considered preferable.

The birth

The environment of the birth is very important in particular because for all couples, the sight of their child is the culmination of years of striving, hoping, and longing.

Fathers are often present during the birth, and, in patients having a Caesarean delivery, a lower-back anaesthetic is used where possible so that both father and mother can enjoy the birth experience.

An above-average proportion of babies have been born by Caesarean section following the test-tube procedure. The reasons for this vary.

Patients are generally older than usual, and a long history of infertility may persuade the obstetrician not to take the risk (of oxygen deprivation) of a normal vaginal delivery.

Sometimes there may be complications independent of the procedure that warrant a Caesarean delivery. For example, some women have had previous tubal surgery during which the tube has been joined to the uterus. The risk of a scar's rupturing during labor may influence a decision about the safest method of delivery.

There is little doubt that for the first few test-tube babies delivered parents and doctors were extremely anxious, and this may have contributed to decisions in favor of Caesarean deliveries. Since these early births, a considerable number of babies have been born by the normal vaginal route and it is almost certain that, in the future, most test-tube babies will be born in this way.

After birth, babies are examined by a pediatrician, and mothers and babies remain in the hospital until both are well and the baby's feeding routine is established.

Post-natal depression

There is a high level of excitement associated with pregnancy and birth following the test-tube-baby procedure, and it is to be expected that many mothers will experience a let-down feeling, often described as "the baby blues," after the birth. Understanding and support from partners, relatives, friends, and counselors is vital.

Additional strain may arise following the birth because of the great interest of relatives and friends. As one father remarked, "It seemed that many people came just to see whether the baby had a glass bottom."

8

How Successful
Is the Procedure?

The success rate of the test-tube-baby procedure can be expressed in several different ways. Some clients quote the success rate in terms of pregnancies per embryo transfer; others present results in terms of pregnancies per laparoscopy.

The first figure gives a higher success rate than the second because it neglects to take into account the failure to pick up any eggs at laparoscopy, unsuccessful fertilization, or abnormal embryo growth. A success rate based on pregnancies per embryo transfer thus gives an overly optimistic picture. In order to provide couples with a more realistic guide to the likelihood of success with the test-tube procedure, it is best to talk in terms of pregnancies per laparoscopy.

In our own clinic, and in successful clinics in the United States and England, this figure varies from 12 to 25 percent. The success rate can alter, even from month to month within the same clinic, for reasons that are not always clear.

It may be that a new member of the team is doing things a little differently, or there may be a new batch of chemicals that is making the culture fluid marginally better or worse. Or a procedure may be altered slightly, and this may have a significant effect on the overall success of the procedure.

During the 1970s, our success rate was very close to zero. But from June 1980 to February 1981, nine pregnancies of more than twelve weeks' duration resulted from 112 laparoscopies, giving a success rate of 8 percent. Because a small number of the pregnancies miscarried after twelve weeks, the liveborn rate per laparoscopy was a little less than 8 percent.

From the program's inception until the end of August 1983, 140 pregnancies occurred among couples joining the Monash/QVMC/

Epworth program. Of these, seventy-five had resulted in live births.

As stated, the pregnancy rate per laparoscopy is about 15 percent. If three treatments are carried out, the chance of a pregnancy is at least 45 percent.

Among the 140 pregnancies there were eight sets of twins and four sets of triplets, so the chance of twins may be five or more times that following conventional conception.

In assessing where improvements in the procedure may occur in the future, it is helpful to look at the success rate of each of the steps involved. In general, the success rate of laparoscopy is more than 90 percent. That is, of ten women who have a laparoscopy, nine will have at least one egg picked up.

In the second step, insemination, fertilization occurs in 80 to 90 percent of couples who have had a laparoscopy. That is, nearly all eggs picked up are fertilized in the laboratory.

However, the embryos so formed may not have a normal appearance, or they may grow very slowly. Of the eggs collected from ten women, embryo growth is normal in six to eight of the ten. The reason for this variation from six to eight is that errors may occur temporarily in the system and when they are corrected, the result may be the higher success rate.

In the final step, embryo transfer, of ten women who have a laparoscopy, only one or two will have a continuing pregnancy. Some of the embryos do not implant; others miscarry. The miscarriage rate in this group was about one in four, but this has decreased to the miscarriage rate among women who have not had IVF and ET (10 to 15 percent) as the quality of embryos has improved.

Why is it that so many embryos that are transferred do not implant? This is the last major hurdle in the procedure, the problem that is puzzling teams in Australia, the United States, and Europe. It may be that some embryos with a normal appearance and growth rate are in some way abnormal and so are aborted naturally.

Another possibility is that the transfer procedure is at fault. But if this is the case, the success rate would not be improved so markedly when transferring several embryos at a time. If, for example, the transfer procedure damaged the embryo, one would expect that whether one or several embryos were transferred, the damage would be done equally and the success rate would vary little if the transfer involved one or more embryos. Analysis of the pregnancies in the Monash/QVMC/Epworth program indicates that if three embryos are transferred there is a 40 percent chance of a continuing pregnancy; if two embryos are transferred, the chance is 28 percent; and if one is transferred, 12 percent.

If, as we suspect, some of the embryos transferred are not completely healthy, then improved methods of assessing embryo health and insights into why the embryo ill health is occurring will be very variable.

It is possible that chemical tests may be developed to distinguish between normal and abnormal (in terms of genetic constitution and development rate) embryos. Preliminary work in this area has been completed in cattle, and application of the findings to humans may be possible. As the quality of the transferred embryos improves, and the miscarriage rate drops, so the success rate of the procedure can be expected to improve.

There is no doubt that because *in vitro* fertilization and embryo transfer are new and rapidly developing procedures in humans, the important matter of success rates has been dealt with arbitrarily—that is, the criteria for defining success were arbitrary. Some groups used the word *success* for achieving fertilization in the laboratory, others for achieving a pregnancy.

It is to be hoped that publicity about programs around the world will quote success rates in terms that do not give infertile couples a distorted and overly optimistic picture. Among a highly selected group of patients, such as those with multiple embryo transfers, the success rate could be artificially elevated. In the Monash/QVMC/Epworth program all patients—many of whom have multiple causes of infertility—are included in the statistical analyses. In the future, couples entering programs can expect more precise statistics that take into account the age and the cause of infertility of patients.

A competitive baby count between different countries or states also may be misleading; couples may have a greater chance of having a baby by working with a highly efficient small team than with a large group whose results look good only because of the substantial number of patients being treated.

Clearly, the success rate is not just a matter of academic interest for teams attempting to maximize the usefulness of the procedure. It is vital information for governments because of decisions about the allocation of health-care resources. And it is crucial for couples because it will undoubtedly influence whether they try for a pregnancy in a local program or enter their names on the waiting lists of programs farther afield.

9
Justification
of the Procedure

The questions most often raised concerning the procedure as currently practiced by the Monash/QVMC/Epworth group are considered in this chapter.

These questions tend to place emphasis on justification of the program rather than on the benefits gained through its use. This is probably a reasonable emphasis as, in general, people assume that we are acting in good faith to assist patients, but they want an assurance that team members are fully aware of the social, ethical, and moral issues involved.

What is the justification for interfering in the natural system of conception?

Medicine has always had the objective of trying to overcome nature's defects. The repair or replacement of parts of the body (limbs, hearts and heart valves, joints, and kidneys) is ample evidence of man's successful efforts in this respect.

Since the time of Hippocrates codes of medical ethics have stressed the doctor's duty to relieve suffering, a variety of which is exemplified by the situation of infertility. And the United Nations Declaration of Human Rights (Geneva, 1948) affirmed the right of every individual to have a family.

To deny people the objective of trying to overcome nature's errors is to obliterate a substantial portion of current medical practice.

It would seem inconsistent to call for a moratorium on medical assistance that enables or helps men and women create the new life of a child—by treating infertility through the test-tube-baby procedure, with drugs or tubal surgery—without also placing a moratorium on man's interference in preventing or delaying death. Both creation and death are natural, some would say God-directed, processes.

A Jesuit theologian, William Daniel, raises other issues when he says:

> The main ethical problem I have with IVF is whether it is sufficiently respectful of the human life of the embryo.
>
> What I find most disturbing in all this field of reproductive biology is the growing assumption that the will and the power of the adult world shall reach into the life of the child, to give life and to take it away. The perspectives are entirely one-sided, and the assumptions are extremely dangerous.

These are reasonable concerns, and every IVF team has a responsibility to provide clear statements of what is done and why so that others may judge whether there is sufficient respect for the human life of the embryo and whether the new power to assist in the creation of life is considerate of the life of the child.

In this regard, studies are under way to assess the psychological and physical effects of IVF on the child. Conclusive answers will be possible only after many more children have been born following this procedure, and after long-term studies of their development have been conducted.

Until sufficient children have been studied carefully, it seems prudent to restrict the procedure to teams capable of carefully monitoring the pregnancy, birth, and child-rearing period.

How can wastage of embryos be justified?

Wastage is a relative term in reproduction. Nature provides a most effective system whereby many abnormal embryos are lost naturally, usually at a very early stage of development before a woman is aware of a pregnancy. Studies based on blood tests and natural pregnancy rates of fertile populations indicate that between 20 and 55 percent of embryos are lost naturally each cycle.

In 1981, the spontaneous abortion rate (missed period) following IVF and ET was 36 percent in the Monash/QVMC/Epworth program, a figure that was reduced in 1982 to 10 to 15 percent—comparable to the natural situation. The IVF spontaneous abortion rate is likely to appear high because patients are monitored very carefully and their pregnancies are identified at a much earlier stage than are pregnancies established through sexual intercourse.

Both in the conventional situation and following IVF, it is likely that most of the unsuccessful embryos are abnormal (genetically or developmentally) in some way. As the abnormal embryos do not have the potential to develop into human life in the form of a fetus, a baby, or an adult, it is difficult to define their ethical status.

It is interesting to note that religious and legal authorities have not considered seriously the status of early abnormal embryos that abort naturally. Such consideration might lead to the view that there is a moral or legal obligation to preserve them.

The religious status of the embryo is relevant to the viewpoint adopted. Entrapment of the soul in the embryo and fetus is still a matter of debate within Church circles. Some theologians favor the view that the soul enters the embryo at the time of conception; others share the belief reflected in Church teaching before the thirteenth century and by St. Thomas Aquinas, that the soul enters the embryo and fetus in a gradual process.

The latter view dovetails with scientific knowledge concerning embryological development and with the legal distinctions between the fetus, newborn baby, and adult. This viewpoint would also allow for different weight to be given to attempts to preserve life at the stages of embryo, fetus, and newborn baby.

The embryo wastage, but not the abortion rate, is higher with IVF and ET than in the natural situation, but the extent of the difference cannot be estimated because of lack of knowledge about early embryo (unimplanted) wastage under normal conditions.

With the development of the test-tube procedure, it is our hope that improvements can be made that will reduce the embryo wastage rate to a situation comparable to, or less than, that existing under conventional conditions of conception.

Can the cutting up of embryos for research purposes be justified?

In our program, all embryos with a normal appearance and growth rate are transferred to patients or are stored frozen for future use by the couple. If an embryo is abnormal, the IVF team may study it to try to determine the cause of the abnormality. It is thought that because an abnormal embryo is degenerating and will probably soon die, it no longer has the potential for life.

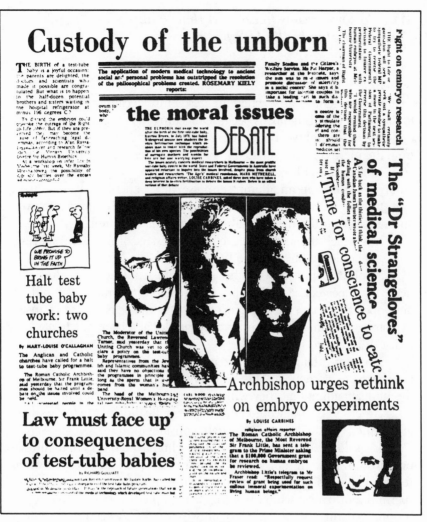

Figure 21.

The definition of embryo death is an uncertain area. It is not possible to use the same criterion as for children or adults—namely, cessation of brain function—in assessing whether an embryo is alive or dead, as brain tissue does not start to form until the embryo is two to three weeks old.

The most reasonable definition of embryo death seems to be when the embryo no longer has the potential for life, and the best indications of this at present are abnormal structure or a slow rate of growth.

99

Why do some teams freeze and thaw embryos and eggs? (Not applicable in the U.S.)

The freezing and thawing of embryos is carried out solely to help overcome infertility.

Circumstances arise when the fresh embryo cannot be transferred to the patient. This happens because bleeding may occur in the uterus, and if a fresh embryo is transferred at this time, it is either washed from the uterus or encapsulated in blood and therefore cannot implant.

In an attempt to save the fresh embryo, two steps are taken. The embryo is frozen in an attempt to preserve it. Then, in a subsequent menstrual cycle, soon after the time of ovulation, the embryo is thawed and replaced in the uterus in the hope that it will implant.

If this technique can be developed to a stage of consistent success, embryos could be saved that otherwise would be lost.

Another application of this procedure would be to reduce the need for repeated egg pick-ups. If three to five embryos could be developed from each pick-up procedure, it would be possible to transfer two embryos immediately and the remainder at a later date to achieve a first or a second pregnancy.

It is not intended that frozen embryos be kept for decades and transferred to women of a different generation. Embryos are frozen on the understanding that they will be transferred to the patient.

An embryo bank would be another application of the freeze-thaw technique, but this requires separate consideration.

Eggs donated by women to others who have no eggs of their own or whose ovaries are not accessible may be frozen and thawed when required. This situation is similar to the use of frozen sperm from sperm donor banks, which has enabled couples to have a child when the male partner is infertile. (In the U.S., the availability of donor sperm and eggs is very limited.)

It is not certain that the freezing and thawing of embryos will succeed in the human, but the indications are that it is technically feasible. Several eight-cell embryos have been frozen at the Queen Victoria Medical Centre that, on thawing, have had a normal appearance and growth. However, as of the middle of 1983, embryos transferred following freezing and thawing have resulted in continuing pregnancies.

Is the test-tube-baby procedure excessively costly?

The financial cost of the program seems to have attracted criticism on the grounds that it is ethically wrong to divert large sums of money and many talented people to a procedure useful to only a small percentage of the population and likely to succeed in no more than 40 to 50 percent of those participating.

It must be remembered that many new medical techniques are expensive at the outset and the cost decreases as the technique becomes routine.

This has been the case with the test-tube procedure. The development of the Monash/QVMC/Epworth program has cost less than $1 million over a decade, a relatively small sum for a research project that has already achieved a significant measure of success.

The cost of the treatment—about $3000 to $8000 for each attempt—is similar to the cost of an operation to repair the Fallopian tubes. Whereas the pregnancy rate following tubal surgery is approximately 30 percent overall, following the test-tube procedure it is approximately 40 to 50 percent after three attempts. Indeed, the IVF procedure is now more cost-effective than tubal surgery carried out when the tubal operation has a 10 to 20 percent chance of success.

As the test-tube procedure has been developed only recently, it is reasonable to assume that with further improvements the cost may be reduced and the success rate increased. After all, the techniques of tubal surgery have been developed gradually over a period of nearly a century. Financial priorities for health care are based on community needs and demand and we would not wish money to be diverted from programs considered to be more important.

Would it not be more useful if the expertise of your group were directed toward developing new contraceptives or trying to discover important causes of fetal malformation?

The reason for deciding to work in the area of infertility was that in the late 1960s when the project began, the community pressure for treating infertility was stronger than for finding new contraceptives.

When the program started we were not certain that it would result in the achievement of pregnancies, but it seemed reasonable to believe that the basic information acquired from the work might help in the areas of sperm-egg interaction, contraceptive development, and in greater understanding of fetal malformation.

Support for this view came from the Ford Foundation, which provided a five-year grant to the project on the grounds that the information gained would be useful in future contraceptive research. Some of the information from our work has been used already by

101

research scientists in an attempt to develop a contraceptive vaccine that would prevent sperm cells from entering the egg.

For infertile couples, the benefits of the program include the prospect of overcoming infertility, a diagnosis of its cause, alleviation of any feeling of guilt that may have arisen as a result of previous venereal disease or abortion, exploration of every available avenue to become pregnant, and the satisfaction of collection of a normal egg or of development of a normal embryo, even if not pregnancy.

The benefits to society are several. Infertility may be resolved for many thousands of couples, new causes of infertility are being discovered, and increased knowledge concerning human fertilization may result in the development of new contraceptives as well as provide insights into ways of reducing birth defects.

How can the program be justified in view of Church criticisms?

In Australia, criticism of the procedure has come mainly from some leaders of the Roman Catholic and Anglican Churches, but not all ordained or lay members of these churches agree with these opinions.

A Gallup poll conducted in the United States after the birth of Louise Brown in 1978 found that 56 percent of Catholics approved of the procedure. A comparable percentage of Australian Catholics polled in 1981 also approved of the procedure as practiced in Melbourne.

And the Anglican Church's social responsibilities commission has agreed that "IVF may be ethically acceptable in the case of childless married couples who cannot have children by any other means."

Church criticism has centered on embryo wastage, the freezing and thawing of embryos, dissection of early embryos, and the possibility that the procedure may lead to other types of research such as cloning, gene engineering, and the creation of hybrids. Although the first two of these areas (embryo wastage and the freeze-thaw procedure) are necessarily involved in our approach, the third and fourth (embryo dissection and manipulation) are not taking place and need not occur in the future if the community finds them unacceptable.

It is worth remembering also that many people do not approach the resolution of the ethical problems raised by the procedure from the perspective of a clearly defined moral position. Surveys in Australia, and the answers to the national census, suggest a decline both in association with organized religion and in church-going. This situation cannot be ignored when responding to complex ethical issues and to the appeal for their solution by reference to Church teachings that are not generally—let alone universally—accepted.

What does the community think?

Results of opinion polls in the United States and in Australia indicate that the majority of people favor the test-tube-baby procedure for helping married couples who cannot otherwise have children.

A survey conducted in June 1981 by an independent public opinion research center (Roy Morgan, Australia) that involved interviewing a cross-section of 1000 men and women aged fourteen and over found that 77 percent approved of the method, 11 percent disapproved, and 12 percent were undecided. In July 1982, the approval rate was 72 percent. Recent polls in the United States indicate comparable figures. Age and educational level are the main factors affecting acceptance, with those aged over seventy and those with a primary (elementary) school education most likely to disapprove. This is true in both countries.

Most people who approved said that the program gave all people the opportunity to have children. Others said, "The decision is up to the parents," "It is the only way for some couples; adoption is difficult," or "It brings happiness into people's lives."

Of those surveyed in Australia, only 1 percent in the first survey and 2 percent in the second opposed the procedure on religious grounds. A 1978 Louis Harris poll in the United States revealed that 30 percent of respondents who disapproved did so on moral and religious grounds.

In Australia a small group—5 percent in the first survey and 6 percent in the second—opposed it on the grounds that it is not natural. The 1978 Harris poll, however, found that almost half of those who opposed the procedure did so because "it is unnatural." Interestingly, more than half of those who disapproved of the program could not say why they disapproved. This suggests uncertainty about what IVF might lead to in the future rather than a specific current problem.

Aren't you and your colleagues playing God?

Teams involved in test-tube-baby programs do not make life; they assist in creation by using God's materials—the sperm cells of the male, the egg of the woman, and the brains and skills of scientists, doctors, and many others.

Working in such a program tends to increase wonderment and admiration for the creative process. If one believes that God created man, the work would seem to be pro-, not anti-, religious.

If God's will is that man should be created by the act of bodily love, which is absent in the test-tube-baby procedure, how can the procedure be justified?

According to some authorities, bodily love was not involved in the creation of the founder of Christianity, Jesus Christ, since his mother was a virgin. It therefore seems inconsistent to insist that bodily love is such a necessary part of human creation.

Furthermore, the act of bodily love is not necessarily linked with procreation. Bodily love occurs between couples for many reasons other than to have children: for pleasure, erotic satisfaction, leisure, or even habit. And the Church makes no objection to bodily love at times when the couple are not fertile—indeed, this is a church-favored method of birth control.

Love between married couples—whether they are fertile or in-fertile—incorporates the mind and the body. Partners taking part in the program are not less in love and, indeed, may express their love for each other more strongly than in the natural system by making considerable personal sacrifices.

If opposition from the Churches threatens the continuation of the program, how can this be resolved?

One way of resolving differences of opinion within the community would be to have an agency to set guidelines and oversee such programs. The views of churchmen and women, lawyers, health professionals, and other groups and individuals in the community who wish to have their opinions considered could then be presented, and it would probably be possible to reach a consensus on acceptable practices.

Suitable guidelines need to be laid down by government authorities to ensure that the techniques involved are not used in unacceptable types of experiments, and already the groundwork is being laid for achieving such a consensus. The Parliament of the Australian state of Victoria has formed a committee to explore the social, ethical, and biological implications of the procedure, and Australian national bodies examining the implications of the work include the National Health and Medical Research Council, which in August 1982 officially approved IVF and ET, including the use of donor sperm cells and eggs (see Appendix), and the Australian Medical Association. In the United States, the ethics committee of the National Institutes of Health has studied the issue, as have committees of the Congress.

Does the experimental nature of the procedure expose children who will be born as a result of it to an undue risk of malformation?

This is an area of concern. However, on the basis of the 120 or so children brought into being with the help of IVF and ET up to the middle of 1983, there is no evidence that the procedure causes an above-normal incidence of birth defects (see Chapter 7). Indeed, the 3 percent rate of major malformations in the children of couples who are reproducing without the help of IVF suggests that the procedure may actually *reduce* the risk of birth defects. The same procedure in several other species has resulted in a normal incidence of malformation also.

Theoretical reasons might lead one to suspect that the risk of malformation would be somewhat different from what it is in normal circumstances. For example, because a large number of sperm cells are placed with the egg, more than one sperm might enter, resulting in a chromosomal abnormality. Fortunately, this occurrence usually results in poor fertilization, failed fertilization, or very early embryonic death. During the past thirty years there has only been one surviving baby in the state of Victoria that was possibly created as a result of more than one sperm cell's entering the egg. This baby had multiple malformations and died on the day of birth.

Couples are informed about the possibility of malformation and the evidence for and against this possibility. The couples make the decision about whether to proceed with the treatment, and, should a pregnancy result, tests to detect malformation are offered.

It should be remembered that procreation by orthodox methods produces deformed and defective children, yet no one suggests a ban on sexual intercourse.

In the future it may be possible for the test-tube-baby procedure to reduce the incidence of, or eliminate, certain defects from the population. For example, where both partners are carriers of recessive genes that in combination would result in a major birth defect, it may be possible to select eggs and sperm cells that would avoid such a situation (see Chapter 10).

How many therapeutic abortions within the Australian/Melbourne test-tube-baby programs have been required after the embryo has become a fetus?

None. Definite figures for other programs are not available, but as of late 1983 no therapeutic abortions have been reported.

Is not the test-tube-baby procedure likely to result in a "stud farming mentality" that displaces normal sexual relations?

One source of this and similar arguments is the claim of Pope Pius XII that artificial insemination using the husband's sperm cells (AIH, which is used when the husband cannot ejaculate) is immoral because the child so born is not the result of an act that is, of itself, the expression of personal love. To reject this claim is to turn "the domestic hearth, sanctuary of the family, into nothing more than a biological laboratory."

The fallacy of this argument is that the procedure in no way takes place at the expense of normal sexual enjoyment. The procedure is a way of helping partners fulfill their desires to become parents, and, although it requires certain technical procedures, it does not mean that the partners' enduring sexual union takes on the character of a biological laboratory.

Indeed, the Church is quite happy for some technology to enter the bedroom—for example, thermometers used in the Roman Catholic Church–approved Temperature Method of family planning; yet there is no suggestion that this results in the transformation of the bedroom into a biological laboratory.

10

Future Prospects

Cloning a super-race, test-tube hatcheries, embryonic sex selection—these are some of the developments that have been linked with the test-tube-baby procedure and have fueled debate about its ethical basis and social implications.

The concerns about future developments sometimes extend beyond the world of science fact into science fiction, perhaps reflecting a sense of incredulity at man's increasing ability to share in creation. Until this generation, man has managed to procreate without the intervention of technology, and some people fear that this is about to change markedly.

However, future developments may impart substantial benefits as well as suggest possible risks.

One development that promises to extend the treatment possibilities of the procedure significantly is the separation of more active from less active sperm cells in an attempt to ensure that only the healthiest are added to the egg.

Another related development is the possibility of breaking down the outer coat of the egg by chemical means, thus reducing the number of healthy sperm cells needed to achieve fertilization; this could prove to be critically important in the treatment of patients with low sperm counts.

A further simplification of IVF has been described by Dr. Ian Craft in London. He has placed the sperm cells and egg together for only one hour and then transferred them to the uterus. Two of the thirty-one women became pregnant. The procedure requires minimal laboratory facilities, and fertilization takes place within the mother's body.

punctured using ultrasound (sonar) pictures. Only local anaesthesia is required.

Another important simplification of the technique has been developed that allows eggs to be collected without general anaesthesia and laparoscopy. A needle is passed to the ovary, and the follicles are

Freezing of eggs and embryos

The freeze-thaw procedure (see Chapter 3), already established with regard to sperm cells, is undergoing trials with egg cells and embryos.

Egg or embryo preservation by freezing may be considered a future prospect because, as yet, there has not been a pregnancy reported following this procedure. The technique is routine in many animal species and has a relatively high success rate.

Regardless of developments in *in vitro* fertilization, the option to preserve eggs or embryos for patients seems preferable to disposing of them merely because freezing facilities, which would enable their storage for future use, have not been established.

Many situations arise where immediate transfer of embryos is not possible or advisable. These include situations where the patient is ill, bleeding occurs from the uterus, or an embryo transfer through the cervix is unsuccessful.

In addition, the use of fertility drugs has meant that five or more ripe eggs may be collected at laparoscopy. This may result in the formation of as many embryos, which means that the chances of establishing a pregnancy are greater; our studies indicate that if three embryos are transferred, the likelihood of a pregnancy is 40 percent; if two are transferred, 28 percent; and in the case of one embryo, 12 percent.

Together with an increased likelihood of pregnancy, clinics that use fertility drugs face the possibility of producing more eggs and embryos than are required by the patient for immediate transfer. One way to avoid this situation is to limit the number of eggs collected or used to the exact number required for transfer.

This, however, has several disadvantages. The best eggs may be left in the ovary, or, even if collected, they may not be selected for fertilization. Also, ripe egg follicles remaining in the ovary may develop into painful cysts.

Not using mature eggs may even amount to wasted opportunity. At present it is impossible to identify with any certainty those eggs that will develop into normal embryos. If six eggs are collected, three or four may fertilize and develop normally, but it is possible that more or less than this number will do so.

To provide patients in our program with the greatest possible chance of pregnancy, all the eggs collected are fertilized, and the number of embryos requested by the patient is transferred immediately. Any embryos not transferred at this time are preserved for the couple by freezing until they can be accepted. This is usually within a few months if a continuing pregnancy does not result from the immediate transfer of embryos, or some time later, if there is a successful pregnancy.

If the best eggs could be identified by microscopic examination and/or other tests, freezing would not be required. But in the absence of this capability, we regard attempted freezing as an ethical obligation (see Chapter 9).

Can freezing succeed?

The pre-freezing structure of the embryos has been retained after thawing, and embryos have continued to develop for a further day following culture in the laboratory.

Transfer of thawed embryos and eggs is under way to see if pregnancies can be established.

In the case of either extra embryos or inappropriate conditions for transfer, patients usually prefer to have them frozen, although in an increasing number of cases they have volunteered to donate them to other couples.

In the event of embryo freezing, couples sign a special consent form in which they agree to make the decision as to the ultimate fate of the frozen embryos; and they state their understanding that there is no guarantee of survival of the embryos after thawing.

Some people have suggested that the freeze-thaw technique could be used for the development of procedures such as cloning, but there is no necessary association between the two.

Whether freezing can be applied to the establishment of embryo banks or surrogate pregnancies will depend on the success of the freeze-thaw procedure and advice from committees established to set guidelines for the work (see Appendix).

Donation of embryos (adoption at conception)

Donor embryos are the product of another couple's sperm cell and egg.

The donation of embryos by one couple to another can be seen as a form of adoption in which the adoption occurs at conception, not after birth. Compared with conventional adoption, it would have the advantage that the adoptive couple would experience the pregnancy and birth of the child. A condition of the donation is that the first couple must agree not to make any claims to the child.

The prospect of a continuing pregnancy following transfer of a donor embryo would seem to be favorable, because fetal tissue appears to be protected from the rejection reactions that typically occur when organs are transferred between children and adults.

The transfer of a donor embryo could be considered when:

* adhesions and pelvic disease prevent access to the ovaries.
* complete infertility results from an early menopause, or when the removal or dysfunction of the ovaries results in an absence of eggs. (In such cases, an alternative to a donor embryo would be to fertilize a donor egg with the male partner's sperm cells.)
* the child is likely to be born with a genetic disorder as a result of the combination of the couple's genetic material.
* both a wife and husband are infertile.

Embryo donation could take place after thawing of a frozen embryo, or it could involve the transfer of a fresh embryo.

If a fresh embryo were donated, it would be necessary to synchronize the menstrual cycles of the donor and recipient women. This can be achieved by hormone therapy.

If the donor embryo were preserved by freezing, it could be transferred when the recipient's uterus was in a suitable condition to support embryo growth.

Although embryo donations may provide a way for some infertile couples to become parents, they warrant similar ethical and legal consideration as do egg and sperm donation (the latter is already an established procedure in the form of Artificial Insemination by Donor).

Donation of eggs

Egg donation can be considered a future development because this practice is not yet widely established. The procedure is likely to succeed as two early pregnancies occurred in the first few donor egg attempts; and a third pregnancy resulted in the birth of a healthy boy in November 1983.

Early in 1982, the Ethics Committee of the Queen Victoria Medical Centre approved the donation of eggs, provided that the donation was anonymous and that the husband's sperm cells were used to fertilize the donor egg.

In the donor-egg situation, the baby is the product of the husband's sperm cells, a donated egg, and the nourishment and protection of the wife's uterus during the pregnancy.

It has the possible advantage over embryo donation in that half of the genetic makeup of the child would be derived from the infertile couple. For some couples, this would be considered advantageous, but others could regard the donor egg as an intrusion on the marriage or its use as technical adultery and may therefore prefer embryo donation, which is analogous to adoption.

The conditions of infertility that could be considered for egg donation are similar to embryo donation and include:

- congenital absence of ovaries
- loss of the ovaries due to disease or surgery
- premature menopause where ripe eggs are no longer being produced
- severe pelvic adhesions, or an abnormality, that prevent access to the ovaries by laparoscopy, so that it is impossible to obtain eggs from the patient
- inherited genetic disease that is likely to result in birth abnormalities if the woman's own eggs are used. In this case, a donor egg fertilized by the male partner's sperm cells would substantially reduce the risk of a genetic disease, and couples may prefer this option, given that the wife still plays an essential role by nurturing the developing fetus and giving birth to it.

In the Monash/QVMC/Epworth program, eggs are provided by anonymous donors who are undergoing *in vitro* fertilization themselves and who prefer to donate an egg to another woman rather than have them fertilized and extra embryos frozen. Alternatively, volunteers in the fertile population may agree to donate eggs, particularly, for example, if they have an infertile sister or friend.

Surrogate mothers

In the case of surrogate motherhood a couple could draw up a contract with a woman to act as a substitute or caretaker mother, bearing their embryo formed by IVF (using the couple's egg and sperm) during pregnancy. Then, at birth, the child would be handed over to its genetic parents.

This procedure would seem to be technically feasible by virtue of the protection from rejection that fetal tissue, separated from maternal tissue by the placenta, enjoys.

The prospect of a surrogate could arise if a woman could not or did not wish to carry a pregnancy to term. For example, a woman with an abnormal uterus or with no uterus, but with normal ovaries, might consider the surrogate possibility. Likewise, a woman whose health could be threatened by a pregnancy (for example, a woman who suffers from heart disease or who is partially paralyzed) or who has a history of miscarriages might wish to draw up a contract with a surrogate. Fear of pregnancy or conflicting career interests might also lead to consideration of the surrogate option.

The freeze-thaw technique would allow the embryo to be frozen, then transferred to the surrogate at a suitable stage of her cycle.

Alternatively, a fresh embryo could be used if the cycles of the surrogate and the woman from whom the egg is obtained were synchronized by the use of hormones.

The surrogate option would enable a couple to have a child that is totally genetically their own, without the child's mother ever having been pregnant or given birth.

Another possibility would be for the surrogate to be an AID (Artificial Insemination by Donor) recipient. For example, the husband of a patient with absent or inaccessible ovaries or without a uterus would contribute the sperm cells, and the surrogate would provide the egg.

In recent years in Australia a small number of infertile couples have publicly expressed a wish to obtain the services of a surrogate to help them have a child, and several women have said that they would be interested in becoming surrogates. One such woman who wrote to the Queen Victoria Medical Centre expressed her viewpoint thus:

> I have been interested for quite a long time in the idea of surrogate motherhood. I realize it is a very new idea for enabling some childless couples to have children, and I do appreciate the enormous legal and moral problems involved, and the problem of the emotional involvement of the surrogate mother.
>
> I would be very interested in becoming involved in any work or research that may be done in the future. I've looked at myself and my motives for becoming involved in this, and the effect it would have on my

friends and family. I've come through all this still feeling very confident and very interested.

I will give a very brief description of my reasons for being so interested.

My husband and I have four beautiful children, ranging in age from seven years downwards. My pregnancies were uncomplicated; in fact, I was always my most beautiful when pregnant. It was always a very special and exciting time for me. The births of our four children were also without complication.

My heart goes out to couples who have any sort of problem in regard to having children. I know of the enormous, indescribable importance that "having your own family" can be to two people.

When I first heard of surrogate motherhood, my immediate thoughts were, "Goodness, I could do that! I can't cook, I can't play tennis or do tapestries, but I am good at being pregnant and giving birth." This feeling is directly associated with my concern for the other parties involved—the childless couples. For them, to be able to have their own child in this way—well, I can imagine it would make them terribly happy.

In an Australian public opinion poll conducted in mid-1982 by an independent consumer research organization, 32 percent approved of allowing surrogate motherhood through the program, 44 percent disapproved, and 24 percent had no opinion.

Communities may, in the future, come to regard surrogate motherhood as acceptable and commendable, but the ethical and legal implications of surrogacy contracts require careful consideration, and lawyers who have explored the issues find themselves navigating hitherto uncharted waters.

Regulations governing contracts for surrogate motherhood would need to protect the genetic parents, the surrogate mother, and the child. It is not unreasonable to consider situations involving a dispute between the child's genetic mother and the birth-giving mother (the surrogate). The surrogate, for example, might refuse to relinquish the child.

Given the vital contributions of each to the development of the child, it would be extremely difficult to establish grounds for a decision about maternity rights. Who is the "real" mother in such a situation—the genetic mother or the surrogate mother? Or are they joint mothers? For the surrogate option to be practical, a contract or law would need to establish that the mother who at the outset intends to rear the child is the legal mother.

And what would the responsibilities of the surrogate amount to during the pregnancy, insofar as smoking, drinking, or involvement in dangerous activities that could adversely affect the child's development are concerned?

As regards financial aspects—should there be a recommended and/or a maximum fee for a surrogate's services? Who should pay for medical costs during the pregnancy, particularly where complications necessitate a lengthy hospital stay?

These are just some of the difficult questions surrounding surrogacy contracts that would need to be resolved before such agreements became socially acceptable.

Multiple pregnancies

Microsurgery to the embryos of sheep, mice, amphibia, and cows has resulted in identical twins and triplets.

The procedure involves dividing the early embryo and surrounding each portion so formed with an artificial coat made of agar (a gel-like substance) before transfer to the uterus. Each resulting embryo has the same genetic make-up and is of the same sex as the original embryo.

Another possibility is simply to cut an older embryo in half to make identical twins (see Figure 22).

The natural occurrence of identical twins is the result of spontaneous early embryo division. By copying nature—using microsurgery—the chances of conception and twins could be increased in infertile couples.

It has been argued that the adverse consequences of producing identical individuals could include a sense of alienation from a society reproduced in a different way, and a lack of a sense of uniqueness of

Figure 22. Halving of mature embryo can produce identical twins.

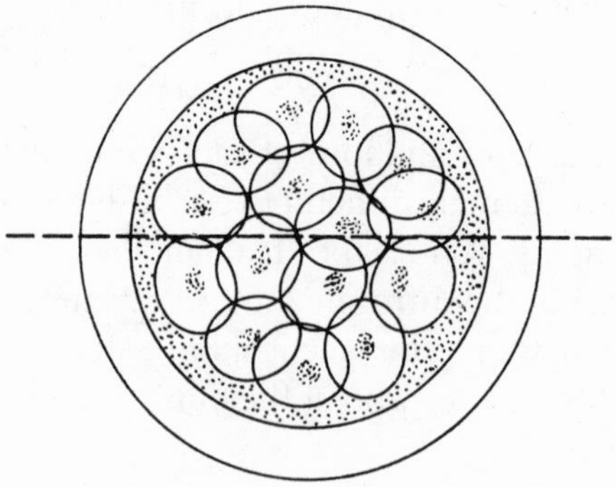

oneself. One would expect a similar alienation to be experienced by children whose existence relied upon artifical insemination, which, like embryo surgery, involves an unconventional method of conception. Yet this alienation has not been reported.

As for a sense of uniqueness, it would seem that identical twins or triplets do not seem to suffer in this way; indeed, they often form very close relationships with one another that are said to be beneficial throughout life. And, given the influence of environment on gene expression, it is doubtful whether the children produced following embryo division would be replicas of each other. This is apparent from identical twins conceived in the orthodox manner—although they are similar in many respects, differences are obvious to those who know them well.

Cloning of embryos

When a sperm cell fertilizes an egg, it achieves two results. First, the introduction of its genetic material; and second, the activation of the egg to divide.

Experiments on mice indicate that it is possible to remove the genetic material of both the fertilizing sperm cell and the egg and replace this with genetic material from another embryo (see Figure 23).

Because embryos contain a number of cells—for example, sixty-four—it is possible to transplant identical genetic material from sixty-four cells to sixty-four activated eggs. The could result in numerous identical offspring that are clones of embryos, not of adults. (Currently, it is not possible to produce completely normal animals after transplanting genetic material from adults.)

Although embryo cloning in this manner may be technically feasible in the human, there seems to be no obvious advantage.

A similar cloning technique has been reported in mice where the nuclei, which contain the genetic material, are taken from an advanced embryo of one hundred cells or more. These nuclei are then injected into eggs after egg chromosomes have been destroyed by ultraviolet light.

Theoretically it would be possible to create up to one hundred clones of one individual embryo if nuclei were obtained from every cell. In practice, very few eggs continue to develop after this procedure of nuclei injection, and consequently very few clones develop to stages of live young.

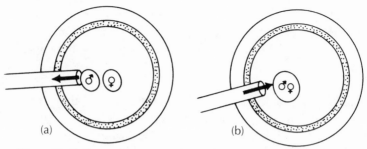

Figure 23. Embryo cloning: (a) removal of genetic material of sperm cell and egg; (b) replacement with genetic material from another embryo.

The prospect of cloning has aroused considerable anxiety, with fears expressed that thousands of Hitlers could be produced. The underlying concern is often the power that such techniques could give to certain individuals to determine the genetic characteristics of future generations. It should be stressed that at present, it is not possible to clone from adult tissues, so duplication of adults is not feasible.

Second, the establishment of a "master race" from cloned embryos would necessitate a captive population of egg and sperm donors and of women to bear the embryos. Given the difficulty, if not impossibility, involved in such scenarios, cloning in human populations seems to be highly improbable.

The fact that selective natural breeding by humans can, and has, achieved master race aims has never been used as an argument against procreation by sexual intercourse.

Micro-injection of sperm cells

As well as current investigations into overcoming the problem of low sperm counts, it may be possible in the future to make use of sperm cells with impaired movement (motility).

This problem may be due to a defect of the sperm "battery," housed within the mid-piece of the sperm cell, that provides energy for movement. Despite this problem, the genetic constitution of the sperm cell may be completely normal.

Under the usual circumstances of conception, such a sperm cell would not be able to fertilize the egg, even if it could reach it, because rapid sperm movement is essential for penetration of the egg.

A future procedure could involve the use of healthy sperm cells from a donor (AID) to pierce the woman's egg and to activate the egg

116

to divide. Then the genetic material of the donor sperm cell could be removed from the egg and replaced with a sperm cell from her infertile partner (see Figure 24). This could have wide application in male infertility.

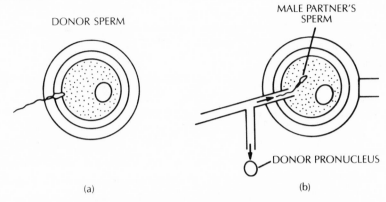

DONOR SPERM

MALE PARTNER'S
SPERM

DONOR PRONUCLEUS

(a)   (b)

Figure 24. Micro-injection technique: (a) healthy sperm cell from donor is used to pierce woman's egg and activate division; (b) genetic material from male partner's sperm replaces donor's.

Another possibility is that micro-injection of an immotile sperm cell would be sufficient to trigger normal fertilization, and therefore the use of donor sperm would not be necessary.

Replacement of male genetic material has been achieved in hamsters.

Injection of genetic material

It is possible to inject sequences of genes (DNA sequences) from rabbits into mouse embryos and to confirm their functional activity in adult mice. This procedure could be adapted for use in humans once the specific DNA sequences missing in various genetic diseases have been identified.

It may then be possible to insert a missing gene (DNA sequence) into the embryo of, for example, a couple known to have a high risk of transmitting a serious genetic disorder.

Sexing of embryos

Determining the sex of the embryo is not feasible at present in the human, but it may become possible in the future.

In animals, embryo sex determination involves the detection of the Y chromosome in cells removed from seven-day-old embryos. Since human embryos of this age are already implanted in the uterus, this procedure is not practical.

If methods could be devised that allowed sex determination of embryos at an earlier stage, the procedure could become feasible. Although it would necessitate the removal of a few cells from the embryo for testing, evidence from animal studies indicates that the embryo would continue to develop normally and would not suffer any defect as a result of the missing cells.

A possible benefit of the sexing procedure would be in situations where the prospective parents are carriers of an inheritable sex-linked disease, such as hemophilia or muscular dystrophy (which affect male offspring only). When it is known that either the female or male children are almost certain to be afflicted, parents may prefer the transfer of embryos of known sex rather than amniocentesis and abortion of a several-months-old fetus. However, female offspring may be carriers of the disease, so the problem could continue in future generations.

Possible medical use of fetal tissue

Currently embryos are not grown longer than five or six days, by which time the blastocyst has distinguishable placental and fetal tissue but no discernible organs.

By about the twelfth day of development, nerve cells and heart tissue have started to form and, as some fetal tissue may not be subject to rejection, it may be feasible to transfer cells from a two- or three-week-old embryo to children or adults who have a disease or abnormality affecting crucial body functions.

It is possible, although unlikely, that the nervous tissue of an early fetus might be capable of overcoming paraplegia or quadriplegia by bridging a gap in the nervous system of the sufferer, pancreatic tissue might be transplanted to overcome life-threatening insulin-dependent diabetes, and fetal kidney tissue might enable kidney function as an alternative to lifelong dialysis or a kidney transplant. It is not known whether transplanted fetal organs would survive, grow, and function effectively.

Whether it is ethical to grow embryos for this purpose should the techniques become feasible in the future needs careful consideration. Serious philosophical, ethical, and moral questions are involved, and it seems appropriate for society to consider these questions because of the very real benefits that these techniques may have for sick or handicapped individuals.

Role of the media in future developments

Whether any or all of these procedures has a future depends on community consensus based on informed discussion. And in this regard, the influence of the press, radio, and television will undoubtedly be extremely important.

Figure 25.

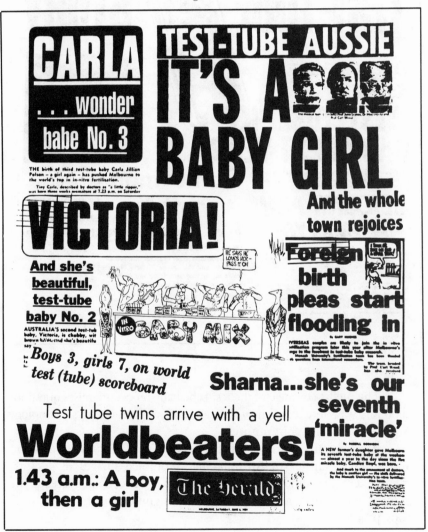

119

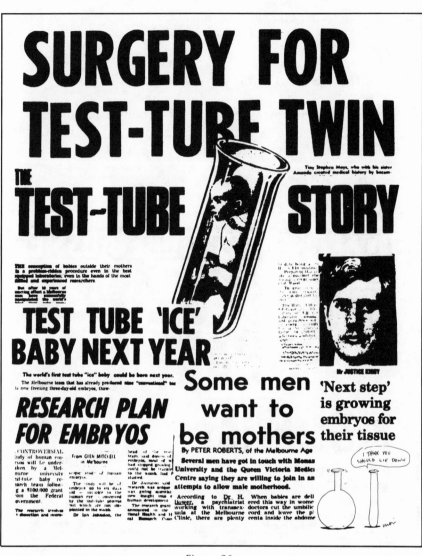

Figure 26.

The media coverage of the test-tube baby procedure raises questions about the ways in which a new, perhaps even a revolutionary, technology is presented to the community.

It has been suggested that the reporting of *in vitro* fertilization and embryo transfer in Australia has promoted images of doctors, infertile couples, and medical science that have helped create the guiding assumptions about the nature and significance of the test-tube-baby program.

Thus one commentator on media coverage of the program remarked:

> The coverage involved a set of paradoxes, a clash of paradigms used to present and explain the story. These centred on: definition of the event (an IVF birth) as a "miracle" while insisting on the "normalcy" of the process; description of infertile couples as a minority group, but using this group to represent all couples; representation of the doctor as a medical authority and father figure.

The temptation to sensationalize—rather than carefully explain—the procedures that may become feasible in the future has been, and will continue to be, a very real problem. As one example, an article in a Melbourne daily newspaper about the freeze-thaw technique, written by a London-based reporter, was to have been headlined: "What the scientists are doing in Melbourne is the most horrifying of all things going on." Before publication, this headline was altered to read "Cloning—and the question that Melbourne raises."

However, the substance of the article failed to produce any evidence of the "horrifying" nature of the Melbourne work, nor did it establish a link between cloning and the test-tube procedure as currently practiced.

There are several difficulties from a journalist's point of view. Translating scientific and technical information into layman's language is a demanding and time-consuming task that requires the equivalent of learning a new dialect. And judging the relevance of the research and gaining a realistic perspective of its implications demands a thorough knowledge of the subject.

Development of IVF clinics

Future developments in IVF and related areas will also have much to do with the success rate of the procedure and the available funds.

Any feasibility study by a clinic contemplating IVF needs to take into account the value of the procedure in treating infertility as well as the technical and staffing requirements of such a clinic.

The manpower requirements include an infertility specialist; an experienced laparoscopist; a reproductive biologist; laboratory technicians for hormone measurements, semen analyses, and preparation of culture fluids, and an ultrasound expert. Other desirable characteristics of a team proposing to do IVF and ET include experience of such procedures in animals, as well as in semen analysis and freezing, infertility assessment, laparoscopy, hormone measurements, and ultrasonic examination. Ready access to operating rooms, tissue culture preparation facilities, a laboratory for quality control procedures, and an ethics committee to set guidelines for the work are also essential.

The barriers to the rapid development of expertise in new groups are numerous, so immediate success is far from guaranteed. For a start, there is still speculation about the factors that contribute to success. And because IVF and ET involve a kaleidoscope of tests, procedures, and technical skills, it is possible that some of the factors contributing to success have not been identified. Variation in our own success rate, when attempting to hold all factors constant, supports this view.

Learning the intricacies of the procedures is the next hurdle. The system is learned best by working with a successful group, but the time available for teaching is limited, and each successful clinic is under considerable pressure to treat as many patients as possible.

As many as one hundred IVF clinics have been established in Europe, the United States, Southeast Asia, and India, and reproduction of the method will become more widespread as teams identify the most important factors in success and simplify the system.

Although it may be feasible to apply some of the procedures described in this chapter, application of the others will be delayed or prohibited either because of the time-consuming and complex nature of the techniques involved or because of ethical considerations.

In deciding upon future directions, the potential benefits of these techniques need to be weighed against the possibility of abuse.

The committees that have been established to investigate the test-tube-baby procedure and its implications are moves toward greater understanding.

We will regard it as a measure of success if readers can understand the essentials of the procedure and can describe it clearly. This is not an impossible dream: Hearing about the birth of twins to a couple in the program, a six-year-old explained the procedure thus:

> The lady had a bend in her pipe that takes the egg to the mother's baby nest. So, the doctor got two eggs from the father's egg factory and they grew into two little tiny babies. Then the doctor put them back in the mother's baby nest and they grew into twin babies.

It is our hope that this book will bring the issues into sharper focus and provide a springboard for well-informed discussion and decision making.

122

Appendix

The following is the August 1982 statement of the National Health and Medical Research Council of Australia officially approving the use of IVF and ET.

In vitro fertilization and embryo transfer

In vitro fertilization (IVF) of human ova with human sperm and transfer of the early embryo to the human uterus (embryo transfer, ET) can be a justifiable means of treating infertility. While IVF and ET is an established procedure, much research remains to be done and the NH & MRC Statement on Human Experimentation should continue to apply to all work in this field.

Particular matters that need to be taken into account when ethical aspects are being considered follow.

1. Every center or institution offering an IVF and ET program should have all aspects of the program approved by an institutional ethics committee. The institutional ethics committee should ensure that a register is kept of all attempts made at securing pregnancies by these techniques. The register should include details of parentage, medical aspects of treatment cycles, and a record of success or failure with: (a) ovum recovery; (b) fertilization; (c) cleavage; (d) embryo transfer; and (e) pregnancy outcome. These institutional registers, as medical records, should be confidential. Summaries for statistical purposes, including details of any congenital abnormalities among offspring, should be available for collation by a national body.

2. Although IVF and ET as techniques have an experimental component, the clinical indications for their use—treatment of infertility within an accepted family relationship—are well established. IVF and ET will normally involve the ova and sperm of the partners.

3. An ovum from a female partner may either be unavailable or unsuitable (*e.g.*, severe genetic disease) for fertilization. In such a situation the following restrictions should apply to ovum donation for embryo transfer to that woman: (a) the transfer should be part of treatment within an accepted family relationship; (b) the recipient couple should intend to accept the duties and obligations of parenthood; (c) consent should be obtained from the donor and the recipient couple; (d) there should be no element of commerce between the donor and recipient couple.

4. A woman could produce a child for an infertile couple from ova and sperm derived from that couple. Because of the current inability to determine or define motherhood in this context, this situation is not yet capable of ethical resolution.

5. Research with sperm, ova, or fertilized ova has been and remains inseparable from the development of safe and effective IVF and ET; as part of this research, other important scientific information concerning human reproductive biology may emerge. However, continuation of embryonic development *in vitro* beyond the stage at which implantation would normally occur is not acceptable.

6. Sperm and ova produced for IVF should be considered to belong to the respective donors. The wishes of the donors regarding the use, storage, and ultimate disposal of the sperm, ova, and resultant embryos should be ascertained and as far as is possible respected by the institution. In the case of the embryos, the donors' joint directions (or the directions of a single surviving donor) should be observed; in the event of disagreement between the donors the institution should be in a position to make decisions.

7. Storage of human embryos may carry biological and social risks. Storage for transfer should be restricted to early, undifferentiated embryos. Although it may be possible technically to store such embryos indefinitely, time limits for storage should be set in every case. In defining these time limits account should be taken both of the wishes of the donors and of a set upper limit, which would be of the order of ten years, but which should not be beyond the time of conventional reproductive need or competence of the female donor.

8. Cloning experiments designed to produce from human tissues viable or potentially viable offspring that are multiple and genetically identical are ethically unacceptable.

9. In this, as in other experimental fields, those who conscientiously object to research projects or therapeutic programs conducted by institutions that employ them should not be obliged to participate in those projects or programs to which they object, nor should they be put at a disadvantage because of their objection.

Glossary

Abortion: The spontaneous or induced termination of pregnancy before it is possible for the fetus to survive outside the womb.

Adhesion: A fibrous band of tissue that abnormally binds organs or other body parts.

Amniocentesis: The puncture of the fluid sac surrounding the developing fetus to obtain a sample of amniotic fluid for testing. The procedure is used to diagnose certain genetic and metabolic abnormalities of the fetus at an early stage of pregnancy.

Artificial insemination: The placement of semen in the vagina, cervix, or uterus by means other than sexual intercourse.

Conceive: To become pregnant.

Conception: The fusion of the egg and sperm cell.

Cyst: Any sac-like structure containing fluid or semi-solid material.

Egg (ovum): The female cell from the ovary that, when fused with a sperm cell, can develop into a new individual.

Ejaculation: Discharge of the semen from the penis.

Embryo: The initial stages in the formation of a new individual in the uterus. In humans, the term is usually restricted to the stage of development from fertilization until the end of the eighth week of pregnancy.

Embryo Transfer (ET): The transfer to the uterus of an early embryo that has been undergoing development in the laboratory.

126

Endometriosis: A condition caused by the presence of pieces of the inner lining of the uterus in areas other than their normal location.

Fallopian tube: The muscular tube along which an egg travels from the ovary to the uterus, and in which the egg is fertilized.

Fertility: The ability to reproduce.

Fertilization: The fusion of an egg and sperm cell.

Fibroid: A fibrous growth of tissue in the muscular walls of the uterus.

Fetus: The developing baby within the uterus. The term describes the embryo from the end of the eighth week of pregnancy until birth.

Follicle: A small fluid-filled structure within the ovary that contains the developing egg. At ovulation, the follicle breaks through the surface of the ovary and the egg is released.

Genetic: Having to do with hereditary characteristics.

Hormone: A chemical substance produced within the body that stimulates or affects organs or other body parts.

Idiopathic infertility: Infertility of unknown cause.

Implantation: The embedding of the fertilized egg in the lining of the uterus.

Infertility: The inability to conceive or reproduce.

In Vitro Fertilization (IVF): Fertilization outside the body in laboratory glassware. "In vitro" means literally "in glass."

Laparoscopy: A procedure in which a combination eyepiece and light is passed into the abdomen or pelvis to enable visual inspection of the internal organs. In IVF, the procedure makes possible the collection of eggs.

Masturbation: Stimulation of the sexual organs to produce sexual release.

Menstrual cycle: The cycle of events occurring regularly in women's reproductive organs during their fertile years. The cycle is most apparent when the lining of the womb is shed at approximately monthly intervals resulting in blood loss from the vagina over a series of days.

Ovulation: The release of the egg from the ovary.

Semen: The sperm-containing fluid released by a man during intercourse or masturbation.

Sperm: The male reproductive cell that, on fusion with the egg, can develop into a new individual.

Ultrasound: A diagnostic technique that uses sound-like waves to produce an image of internal body structures.

Index

130

physiologic changes during, 6
timing of, 5
Intrauterine device (IUD), 14
In vitro fertilization (IVF), 1–2, 32–33, 47–49,
  54–55
  anxiety about, 85–86
  clinics, 121–22
  development of technique, 42–46
  ethics of, 96–97
  National Health and Medical Research Council of
    Australia statement on, 123–25
  procedure of, 69–70
  spontaneous abortion rate following, 97–98
  success rate of, 94
  (*see also* Test-tube-baby program)
Isolation response, 33–34
IVF (*see In vitro* fertilization)

Johnston, Ian, 41

Kremer test, 26
Kretser, David de, 42

Laparoscopy:
  egg pick-up by, 42, 63–66
  infertility diagnosis with, 23–25, 48
  success rate of, 94
  surcharge for, 83
Lawson, R., 42
Leeton, John, 41
Legal protection, 87–88
Lopata, Alex, 41–43
Luteinizing Hormone (LH), 10, 24, 31, 61–62

Marijuana, infertility and, 18
Marital stability, 55, 85
Masturbation for semen collection, 21–22, 68,
  86–87
Media, role in future developments, 119–21
Menstruation, 10
Micro-injection of sperm cells, 116–17
Microsurgery, 39–40
Miscarriage, 78
Monash University Infertility Service, 45, 78, 83, 93–
  96, 101, 111
Mongolism, 89–90
Moore, Neil, 41
Morgan, Roy, 103
Mucus scores, 60
Mucus–sperm incompatibility, 26
Multiple pregnancies, 114–15
Mumps, 21

**National Health and Medical Research Council of
  Australia, 123–25**
Needle biopsy, 22

Obese patients, 51
Obstetrical complications, 89
Oligospermia, 21
One-cell embryo, 11
Opinion polls, 103
Ova (*see* Eggs)
Ovaries, 9
  accessibility of, 51
  physiologic changes during arousal, 6
Ovulation, 5, 10, 18
  estimation of, 58–59
  as selection requirement, 50–51

Parlodel, 32
Penis, 8–9
Pergonal, 58, 59
Physical causes of infertility:
  in men, 7–8, 20–22, 26
  in women, 22–26
Physician, choice of, 91
Pill, the, 14
Pituitary gland, 9–10
Pituitary hormone, 10, 32
Pius XII, Pope, 106
Polyspermy, 90
Post-coital test, 26
Post-natal depression, 92
Pregnancy, 3–12
  embryonic development, 11–12, 70–73
  fear and anxiety about, 4–5
  implantation of embryo, 11–12, 19, 94
  increasing chances of, 5
  multiple, 114–15
  natural fertilization, 6–12
  in test-tube-baby program, 89–92
Progesterone, 12, 19, 24, 62
Progestogens, 29
Prolactin, 18, 24–25, 27, 32
Prostate gland, 8, 22, 28
Psychological factors:
  in infertility, 27, 28
  during pregnancy, 91
Psychological selection criteria, 52–53

**Queen Victoria Medical Centre, 40–46, 67, 73, 78,
  83, 93–96, 101, 110–12**

Reed, Candice, 43
Relaxation, 52
Religious aspects of program, 102–5
Religious influences on family size, 4
Religous status of embryo, 98
Renou, Peter, 43–44
Roman Catholic Church, 102–3
Royal Women's Hospital, 41–43
Ruben's test, 28–29

Sathananthan, Henry, 44–45
Screening for infertility problems, 19–20
Self-treatment of infertility, 18–19
Semen, 6, 7
  analyses of, 21–22, 51
  collection by masturbation, 21–22, 68, 86–87
  infertility and, 7–8
  (*See also* Sperm cells)
Sexing of embryos, 117–18
Sex ratio of births, 89
Sexual arousal, physiologic changes in, 6, 8
Sexual behavior, 4, 6, 18–19
Sexual counselors, 28
Sexual dysfunction, 6
Sheep experiments, 42–43
Speculum, 75
Sperm cells:
  activity of, 9
  anatomy of, 69
  capacitation of, 11, 68–69
  ejaculation of, 9
  incompatability between female genital tract
    and, 26
  in vitro fertilization by, 69–70

131